# GOING GREEN

## 100's OF MONEY-SAVING IDEAS

**Save Thousands with Simple
Energy-Saving Tips!**

**Including How to Clean Your House
Without Harmful Chemicals**

**by
Randall Earl Dunford**

**Magni**

Website: www.magnico.com

41007120    3/09
ISBN: 978-1-882330-97-3

Manufactured in the United States of America

## NOTICE

This book is designed to provide useful and safe information, and every effort has been made to insure the accuracy of its contents.

Success with using the suggested substances and procedures will depend upon such factors as the hardness of the water, temperature of the water, exact quantities of ingredients used, how dirty the surface is, the condition of the item being cleaned, etc. Therefore, although you will be dealing with capable substances that are not harmful to the environment, there can be no ironclad claim or guarantee by the author or publisher that any cleaning formula will be perfectly effective or 100% safe in every single case.

For instance, undiluted vinegar on a delicate fabric such as silk can result in damage to the material. And borax, although it is considered a mild cleaner compared to many supermarket cleaning products, can be toxic if taken internally. In addition, old stains that have become deeply embedded in certain fabrics may never be totally eliminated.

The wisest measure is to observe all cautions in the pages within, proceed slowly, and remember to never abandon common since.

# CONTENTS

# INTRODUCTION

Let's face it. The cleaning chores must be done. And you need reliable and approachable essentials to do them—without taxing your budget. There are thousands of potent products on the market, all-purpose cleaners as well as ones suited for every possible purpose. If you were to purchase one for each application, however, it would consume more indoor real estate than you would desire. More importantly, it could become quite expensive—and wasteful—since products can be used interchangeably. Besides, certain ones may leak toxic vapors into the air, which, even in small levels, can eventually create allergies and other health problems. Some can also lose their effectiveness over time, especially if improperly stored. Others can cause damage to materials if overused or spilled, affect the skin due to prolonged or undiluted exposure, or be highly poisonous to children if ingested. In addition, what you discard winds up in landfills, which, in turn can seep into the water supply. Ditto for what you wash down your drain.

But there are alternatives that are surprisingly effective for cleaning without resorting heavily to harsh formulas that often come with a higher price tag. That's largely what this book is about. You'll find basic answers for every aspect of cleaning—remedies that are economical, easy to use, and always environmentally friendly, from adding salt to the water for an aid in cleaning dishes to vinegar and vegetable oil for cleaning wood floors. These home brews can actually work just as well, if not better, than major supermarket brands. And you will not only find the formulas, but a list of tools and the procedures for keeping every corner your home in top condition, arranged in user-friendly fashion.

And that's not all! Also included within these pages is a special chapter dedicated to strategies for establishing and maintaining the most efficient household possible. You will discover numerous useful ways to save energy, and that, of course, boils down into *saving* lots of *money!* What do you do about insulation? How do you best deal with your water heater? What about heating and cooling? How do you handle appliances in the most advantageous fashion? Even the latest about lighting and home/office equipment is included, as well as many other helpful tips.

You'll also discover another special chapter that will help you to make your cleaning life easier, while saving even more money. What is the best vacuuming equipment? How about air filtration and air purification? What's the best way to deal with pets? How can you more safely discourage insects?

It's all here—in one neat package. In the end, you will not only have a home that is clean and green, but you will save lots of money as well.

Good luck and happy cleaning.

# Helpful Terms

# A LIST OF TOOLS AND SAFE CLEANING INGREDIENTS

The list in this section is confined largely to the most readily obtainable environmentally friendly materials (those from supermarkets, health food stores, pharmacies and the like.) Many of them are interchangeable, so you don't have to always take every formula to heart and adhere to it strictly. There are some exceptions, however, such as the fact that baking soda, washing soda and borax are not good for aluminum.

Feel free to experiment with the proportions you use. You are not a chemist. Who says you have to painstakingly measure ingredients? It depends on the size and difficulty of the job, your preferences, how hard the water is, etc. Just make sure to observe all cautions in the following pages.

Most of these substances are sufficient in themselves. Baking soda, for instance, contains enough abrasiveness to clean many objects. Vinegar, on the other hand, is acidic and will eat through a lot of stains. If neither one by themselves will take care of a job, combining the two may provide you with the best of both worlds and will increase your chances of conquering your task.

While you're at it, remember to get the most out of everything in time and materials. If you are using lemons for cleaning metal, for example, why not use the ones that have been left over from a meal? Or if you are brewing tea for dinner, make enough to clean the windows if they are due for attention. Or pour the vinegar you have used to clean the coffee pot over your rubber drainboard. (Not only will this clean the drainboard, but the vinegar that drips off it will be good for the drainpipe.)

## Handy Cleaning Tools

**Bowl swab:** A cotton or rayon ball attached to a plastic handle. Used for applying cleaner to your toilet bowl. (Available at janitorial supply houses.)

**Broom:** Familiar to everyone. Avoid using for inside jobs, since it stirs up a lot of dust.

**Dry Sponge:** A dry sponge is made of natural open-cell rubber that comes wrapped in plastic and used by many to clean wallpaper. It is versatile, however, and can be used for most any of your home surfaces. To be discarded when saturated with dirt. Use them for dry cleaning only. Exposing them to moisture will render them useless. (Available at paint stores or janitorial supply stores.)

**Lambswool duster:** Fluffy ball of wool (or sometimes synthetic) attached to a long handle for picking up dust particles by means of static attraction. Especially handy for reaching high and low areas. (Available at housewares stores or janitorial supply stores.)

**Mop:** No one must be without this implement. Just make certain and use it for cleaning with the most environmentally safe substances. (Widely available.)

**Spray bottle:** An inexpensive plastic container with a squeeze trigger. Convenient when dispensing cleaner on stains, bathroom tile, etc. (Available at discount stores or janitorial supply stores.)

**Squeegee:** A T-shaped tool with a rubber blade used largely for washing windows. (Available at supermarkets or janitorial supply stores.)

**Toothbrush:** We all know what these are. Not only can they save the day for your teeth, but they are handy when cleaning less accessible areas such as can openers, jewelry, the spots around faucet handles, or ridges in numerous surfaces.

## Environmentally Friendly Ingredients

**Alcohol:** A number of varieties are useful for removing stains besides rubbing or denatured alcohol, such as vodka and brandy. Denatured or isopropyl alcohol is preferable to the standard rubbing kind because it does not contain excess water or perfumes. Alcohol also serves as a disinfectant. Remember, however, that it is flammable. (Widely available.)

**Alum:** A mineral that is used as an astringent and a natural dye fixative. It is an efficient stain remover that works particularly well with lemon juice or vinegar. (Available in crystal form at supermarkets.)

**Australian tea tree oil:** An essential oil that functions as a mildew inhibitor and a disinfectant. (Available at health food stores.)

**Baking Soda (Sodium bicarbonate):** Also known as bicarbonate of soda. More than just an ingredient in baked foods. It can be used as a substitute for toothpaste, as an antacid, to relieve the pain from burns, as a mild bleach, and to extinguish fires, as well as for cleaning and deodorizing. It neutralizes acid stains. Surprisingly effective. (Available at supermarkets.)

**Beeswax:** A natural, hard wax originating from bees. It possesses a rich and unique fragrance. (Available at art stores and furniture-making supply houses.)

**Borax:** A natural, all-purpose powdered cleaner composed of boron, sodium, oxygen and water that is recommended for everything from clothes washing to cleaning the bathroom tile. Serves as a bleach, detergent, deodorizer, disinfectant, mildew retardant and water softener. It is toxic if taken orally. (Available at supermarkets.)

**Chalk:** An opaque white mineral that can be used as a cleaner or whitener. (Available at hardwares stores.)

**Charcoal:** Functions as an excellent odor absorber. (Charcoal blocks are widely available.)

**Club soda:** More than a beverage. It can also be used as a cleaner. (Widely available.)

**Cornmeal:** Meal made from corn. Excellent for a number of cleaning purposes. (Available at supermarkets.)

**Cornstarch:** A starchy flour made from corn and used for cooking. Excellent for many cleaning purposes. (Available at supermarkets.)

**Cream of tartar:** A white crystalline mineral used in medicine and for cooking. Has acidic properties. Functions as a cleaner for metal, toilets, etc. (Available at supermarkets.)

**Flour:** Serves as an abrasive in environmentally friendly cleaning formulas. (Widely available.

**Fuller's earth:** A mixture of alumina and silica that can be used as an absorbent when cleaning. (Available at drug stores.)

**Glycerin:** An odorless, colorless liquid used, among other things, as a solvent and a skin lotion. Functions as a good stain remover. (Available at pharmacies and health food stores.)

**Hydrogen peroxide:** A colorless liquid used for cosmetic, medicinal, and other purposes. Sold in a dilute solution of approximately 3 percent. It will lift certain stains from fabrics. (Available at pharmacies.)

**Kitty litter:** Can be used as an absorbent when cleaning voluminous spills. (Widely available.)

**Lemon juice:** As far as environmentally friendly cleaning is concerned, one could almost accomplish all that is needed with nothing more than a lemon tree in the backyard. Lemon is one of your best friends when it comes to cleaning because it does most of the work for you. Its high acidic content eats deep into dirt and stains. Other citrus fruits function in the same way but are somewhat less potent because their acidic content is slightly lower. (Widely available.)

**Lemon oil:** Can be used instead of fresh lemons or lemon juice. (Available at supermarkets.)

**Linseed oil:** A yellowish oil derived from flaxseed. Because of its fast drying time, it is used in many compounds. Beware of linseed-oil products available in hardware or paint stores. They may contain petroleum products, which can emit toxic vapors when heated. Seek food-grade linseed oil at a health food store.

**Mineral oil:** Although a petrochemical product, this odorless oil is relatively safe to use. (Available at drugstores.)

**Olive oil:** Oil extracted from olives, which is used in cooking. Excellent for polishing wood. (Available at supermarkets.)

**Pennyroyal:** The oil derived from a hairy plant of the mint family. Can be mixed with cleaning formulas to repel fleas. Don't use, however, if pregnant.

**Potter's clay:** Can be used as an aid when cleaning up major spills. (Available at art stores.)

**Pumice:** A porous, spongy stone produced from volcanos. Contained in numerous commercial cleaning powders, it works well for scouring and polishing. It can be obtained in bar or powdered form in various grades of fineness. Not for use on tubs, tile and brightly colored fixtures. (Available at hardware, paint and janitorial supply stores.)

**Rottenstone:** Although the name does not sound very appealing, the powder derived from this soft stone can be used as a metal cleaner and is often effective for removing minor blemishes from furniture. (Available in paint stores.)

**Salt:** Used as a seasoning and preservative. It is a capable, non-scratching abrasive. (Widely available.)

**Sawdust:** Can be used as an absorbent when cleaning serious spills.

**Shampoo:** Can be of assistance in removing some fabric stains. For shampoo containing the most environmentally friendly ingredients, check health food stores.

**Silica gel:** A form of silica used as a drying agent. Discourages mildew by absorbing excess moisture from the air of your home. (Available at camera stores.)

**Sodium percarbonate:** A natural bleach containing hydrogen peroxide and borax. Can be used for bleaching white items. (Available at health food stores.)

**Sodium perborate:** Another natural bleach similar to sodium percarbonate. (May be available at some drugstores. Also, see "Chemical Supply Companies" in the yellow pages.)

**Toothpaste:** Functions as a mild abrasive. Do not use anything but white toothpaste, however, for purposes of cleaning since colors can cause stains.

**Vegetable-oil-based liquid soaps:** Better for the environment than petroleum-based soaps. A perfectly satisfactory, all-purpose cleaner. (Available at health food stores.)

**Vinegar:** This readily available substance, produced by the fermentation of natural sugars, is useful for cleaning many surfaces. Vinegar is useful because it is acidic like lemon juice and therefore holds the ability to neutralize alkaline stains. If you pour a small amount in a dirty sink or bathtub and listen closely for a moment, you can actually hear it at work. Sometimes you can even see it bubbling. Use *white* distilled vinegar for cleaning, not the colored kind. Colored vinegar can leave stains. Do not use on linen, cotton, silk, wool or acetate fabrics without at least a 50/50 dilution. Will also remove odors. (Widely available.)

**Vitamin C capsules (ascorbic acid):** Just what the doctor ordered for toilet bowls. (Widely available.)

**Washing soda (sodium carbonate):** Known to some as washing crystals or sal soda. It is a mineral that is effective for removing oil and grease. Excellent water softener. Since it possesses caustic qualities, those with sensitive skin may need to wear gloves when cleaning with it. Be advised that it can scratch fiberglass. (Available at supermarkets.)

**Zinc oxide:** A white powder that is used in the manufacture of cosmetics, ointments, rubber wares and other items. It can be used as a cleaner. (Available at pharmacies.)

# Chapter 1

# BRAVING THE BATHROOM

A good place to begin a discussion on specific cleanup chores is the bathroom. Not only does this area of the house collect its share of dirt, but because moisture is so prevalent there, the area is a good place for mildew to grow. And that calls for more intense scrubbing.

## Discouraging Mildew

The less moisture that lingers on surfaces, the less mildew you are going to encounter. One good way to keep moisture down is by having an exhaust fan installed. The building code does not require one if a window is present, but that doesn't matter. These devices are wonderful for removal of excessive dampness not only in the bathroom but in the kitchen and basement as well.

The same goes for a heat lamp. It's capable of quickly drying out the air. Either option is worth considering if you don't already have one. Owning both is even better. If nothing else, keep as much light in the bathroom as possible by allowing the light to remain on for a longer duration and/or by pulling back your window curtains and letting in the sunlight whenever you can.

It's also a good idea to keep a special eye out for leaks. Whenever you're cleaning, keep an eye out for suspicious wet spots under the sink, around the base of the toilet, and along the perimeter of the tub. (You should also check the hoses behind your washing machine, under the kitchen sink, and around anything else that could spring a leak, including the ceiling.)

Don't forget to include the bathmat in your washing load often. It accommodates lots of wet feet and absorbs all that moisture. It's better, by the way, to use mats that are made from cotton or some other natural fiber because the dampness will be better absorbed and, therefore, more of it will be confined to the mat itself—not the surrounding area.

It's a good policy to wipe the surfaces of tubs and shower stalls with a towel after each use. Spread out used towels and stretch out shower curtains to hasten drying. If you have glass shower doors, use a squeegee on them after bathing or showering each day to remove the film of water. It is far better to take these steps than to let mildew take root.

---

❈ **Handy Hint:** A small bag of silica gel (available at camera stores) will absorb excess moisture from the air of your home. When it becomes saturated, it will change color but can be reused after drying it out in the oven.

---

## Saying Goodbye to "Soap Soup"

What an irony. Soap is designed for cleaning—not for cleaning up. But how often have you started to work on the bathroom and have ended up battling that soupy, gooey substance that the bar of hand soap itself has created? Even soap dishes with a hollow bottom that allow the soap to drain have to be cleaned before long.

If you don't want to give up your bar soap, allow it to rest on a folded washcloth or sponge. The washcloth or sponge can be dealt with easier because all you have to do is wring it out periodically.

An even better idea is to purchase liquid soap in a pump bottle or hang a liquid soap dispenser. Or, if you want to avoid scented soap completely, just use a handful of baking soda. That's right—baking soda possesses a reasonable amount of abrasiveness and it leaves your hands with a fresh scent. You may miss the lather, but its absence is no indication that your hands, or any surface, will not be clean.

## Rub-a-Dub-Dub, the Ring in the Tub

The first thing you will require to tackle the tub is a long brush. You will also need a pump spray bottle.

> ❋ **Handy hint:** Use a pump spray with the trigger in front, rather than a plunger on top. It will be more convenient to handle.

As for the cleaning formula, pour 1 cup of hot water into the spray bottle, then add 1/2 teaspoon of borax, 1/4 teaspoon of washing soda, 1/4 teaspoon of liquid soap with a vegetable oil base, and 2 teaspoons of vinegar. (You might like to include 1/8 cup of lemon juice as a scent.) Mix thoroughly. If you need more cleaner, increase each ingredient proportionally.

Besides functioning as an all-purpose cleaner, this recipe can be used for the sink, tub or the tile with excellent results. Simply spray the surfaces, then rinse off with a moist sponge. For a heavy-duty tile cleaner, just use plain washing soda. Place the soda on a moist sponge and scrub the surface. Then rinse thoroughly.

> ❋ **Handy hint:** Sometimes this mixture can cause your sprayer to clog. If this becomes a problem, go lighter on the borax and washing soda.

---

❋ **Handy hint:** There is no need to use pure washing soda for light jobs on tile, because it demands a bigger rinsing effort.

---

In a pinch, fresh lemon by itself can work wonders. Just cut one in half, rub it into stains and rinse. Often it will even take care of light iron rust stains.

For tubs that seem hopelessly stained, make a paste by mixing cream of tartar with hydrogen peroxide. Then scrub with a brush. Or fill the tub with enough water to cover the stained areas, add 2 or 3 cups of borax, and let it sit a few hours or overnight. Finish off by scrubbing, then rinsing—and notice how the surface shines.

---

## Suggested Tub, Tile, and Sink Cleaner 1

• 1 cup of hot water
• 1/2 teaspoon of borax
• 1/4 teaspoon of washing soda
• 1/4 teaspoon of vegetable-oil-based liquid
  soap
• 2 teaspoons of vinegar
• 1/8 cup of lemon juice (optional)

❶ Mix thoroughly in spray bottle
❷ Spray surfaces
❸ Scrub with long brush
❹ Rinse thoroughly with moist sponge

---

## Suggested Tub, Tile, and Sink Cleaner 2

• Washing soda

❶ Place the soda on a moist sponge and scrub
❷ Rinse thoroughly

## Suggested Tub, Tile, and Sink Cleaner 3

• Cream of tartar/hydrogen peroxide paste

❶ Scrub with a brush
❷ Rinse thoroughly

## Suggested Tub, Tile, and Sink Cleaner 4

• 2 to 3 cups of borax
• Tub full of water

❶ Add borax to water
❷ Allow to sit a few hours or overnight
❸ Scrub
❹ Rinse

## Suggested Tub, Tile, and Sink Cleaner 5

• Lemon half

❶ Rub into stains
❷ Rinse thoroughly

> ⊠ **Caution:** Do not allow acidic substances to remain in your bathtub or sink. They can eventually damage porcelain surfaces. Instead, use them to clean, then promptly and thoroughly rinse.

> ❋ **Handy hint:** If you are adept with tools, grab a large wrench and unscrew your shower head. Remove the rubber washer and place the head in a pan of 1 part vinegar and 1 part water. Bring the liquid to a boil and allow to simmer for a few minutes. This is an excellent way to dissolve any mineral deposits that are blocking the holes. For those looking for an easier way, tie a plastic bag filled with vinegar over the shower head and leave overnight, then scrub with a toothbrush.

## Bringing Down the Curtain on Soap Buildup and Mildew

Bathtub rings are not pleasant, but neither is a scummed, mildewed shower curtain. For routine cleaning, vinegar comes to the rescue. Simply scrub the curtain with a vinegar-soaked sponge.

If you are faced with a lot of mildew buildup, try this formula: Make a paste, by combining equal amounts of borax and vinegar (or lemon juice). The quantity you use, of course, will depend on how much cleaning you plan to do. A good number is 1/3 to 1/2 cup of each. Apply with a sponge, then rinse thoroughly. You can also place the curtain in a tub of warm water, then add 1/2 cup borax and 1/2 cup salt. Soak for at least an hour. Do not rinse, however, or your purpose will be defeated. Simply rehang and allow to drip dry.

An adequate cleaning mixture, however, will do nothing to prevent a shower curtain from being difficult to manipulate when scrubbing. One way to overcome this hurdle is to have someone hold the curtain taut while you clean.

But if that takes more effort than you would like, just remove the curtain and throw it in the washing machine. Use the warm water setting and add 1/2 cup of borax. Next, add a cup of vinegar to the rinse cycle. Then run it through one more rinse in which you add a cup of salt. Do not spin dry or rinse. Rehang and allow to drip dry. And while you are at it, don't forget about the window curtains. They best be hung outside, however, to dry.

For those with shower doors, the same formulas mentioned above can be used with equal success. (See the chapter 7 for more detail on cleaning glass.)

---

## Suggested Shower Curtain Cleaner 1

• vinegar

❶ Place vinegar on sponge
❷ Rub on curtain

---

## Suggested Shower Curtain Cleaner 2

• 1 part borax
• 1 part vinegar or lemon juice

❶ Mix 1/3 to 1/2 cup of each
❷ Apply with a sponge
❸ Rinse thoroughly

## Suggested Shower Curtain Cleaner 3

- Warm water
- 1/2 cup borax
- 1/2 cup salt

❶ Place curtain in tub of warm water
❷ Add borax and salt
❸ Soak for at least an hour
❹ Do not rinse
❺ Rehang and allow to drip dry

## Suggested Shower Curtain Cleaner 4

- 1/2 cup borax
- 1 cup vinegar
- 1 cup of salt

❶ Place curtain in washing machine on warm water setting
❷ Add borax
❸ Add vinegar to the rinse cycle
❹ Run through additional rinse and add salt
❺ Do not spin dry or rinse
❻ Rehang and allow to drip dry

## No Need to Sink to the Depths of Despair

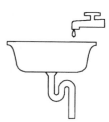

The same formulas used for the bathtub will be just as effective for the bathroom basin. The difficult part is maneuvering around the faucet area, because it's more compact than the bath and shower fixtures. You're lucky if you have single-lever handles, since there will be one less to clean—a fact worth remembering whenever replacing bathroom fixtures. The most effective environmentally friendly combination for plumbing fixtures is 1 part vinegar with 2 parts water. Again, the amount you use will depend on how much cleaning you plan to do. For tough stains, cover the area with a vinegar-soaked tissue and allow it to stay for approximately 5 minutes before scrubbing. Heavy abrasives are not encouraged around this area of the sink (and bathtub) because most faucets contain chrome or nickel plating, and this can wear off.

---

❋ **Handy hint:** Dip an old toothbrush in the cleaning solution and use it in hard-to-reach places. A toothbrush also works well for cleaning the shower nozzle. If necessary, increase the proportion of vinegar.

---

**Suggested Plumbing Fixture Cleaner**

• 1 part vinegar
• 2 parts water

❶ Apply to sponge
❷ Scrub
❸ For tough stains, cover the area with a vinegar-soaked tissue and allow to remain for at least 5 minutes before scrubbing

## Tackling the Toilet

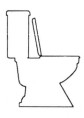

When it comes to that dreaded affair of cleaning the toilet(s), a number of formulas can be put to use that are both easy on the indoor environment and your lungs.

Baking soda is a good stand-by. Just pour approximately half a cup into your toilet bowl and begin scrubbing with your brush.

---

### Suggested Toilet Bowl Cleaner 1

• 1/2 cup Baking soda

❶ Pour into toilet bowl
❷ Scrub with brush
❸ Flush

---

If you are looking to save elbow grease (and who isn't?), use borax instead. Pour in a full cup and let it sit overnight. All you will have facing you the next day is a mild scrubbing job. Borax also doubles as a disinfectant.

---

### Suggested Toilet Bowl Cleaner 2

• 1 cup borax

❶ Pour into bowl
❷ Let it sit overnight
❸ Scrub with brush
❹ Flush

For faster action, add 1/4 cup of lemon juice or vinegar to the borax. Your bowl should be ready for scrubbing within a few hours.

---

**Suggested Toilet Bowl Cleaner 3**

• 1 cup borax
• 1/4 cup of lemon juice or vinegar

❶ Pour into bowl
❷ Allow to sit a few hours
❸ Scrub with brush
❹ Flush

---

Cream of tartar also works in the toilet. Try adding several teaspoons, scrub, and flush.

---

**Suggested Toilet Bowl Cleaner 4**

• 2 or 3 teaspoons cream of tartar

❶ Add to bowl
❷ Scrub with brush
❸ Flush

---

And here's one you won't believe. Take a couple of vitamin C capsules (1000 milligrams), open and drop in. Let the contents sit overnight. The next morning, all you will have to face is a light brush and one flush.

---

**Suggested Toilet Bowl Cleaner 5**

• 2 1000 milligram vitamin C capsules

❶ Open capsules and drop into bowl
❷ Let contents sit overnight
❸ Scrub with brush
❹ Flush

---

If you are battling stubborn accumulations, don't dilute your cleaning formula by pouring it in the water. Use a bowl swab and rapidly push it up and down toward the bottom of the toilet. (A plunger will do in lieu of a swab but it will be difficult to avoid sloshing water onto yourself.) This maneuver will temporarily force the water out of the bowl. Then you can use the swab to apply your cleaner to the exposed surface. It should sit at least several minutes before scrubbing. Flush, and repeat if necessary.

Toilet bowl brushes and swabs should be promptly washed after use with vegetable-oil-based soap and hot water, rinsed well, and hung to dry.

In the event you are left with an unusually stubborn ring around the bowl, a pumice stone or a fine grade sandpaper will almost always remove it. Just make certain the surface is good and wet to prevent the bowl from getting scratched.

---

**Suggested Toilet Bowl Cleaner 6**

• Pumice stone or fine grade sandpaper

❶ Wet surface if necessary
❷ Rub carefully

---

Don't forget the other areas of the toilet. The portion under the rim of the bowl is easy to neglect, as is the rear base and territory under the tank. These areas are excellent breeding grounds for mildew and bacteria. Actually, the base, the seat and other exterior portions of the toilet, as well as under the rim, tend to be more unsanitary than the bowl itself. Bacterial growth there is retarded because of the presence of the cold water.

Before leaving the subject, it is worthwhile to note that you should save the toilet for last to be cleaned. That way any bacteria that is not destroyed when disinfecting will not be inadvertently transferred to tub or sink faucets.

---

❋ **Handy hint:** Even if you have nothing else available at the moment, remember that one of the best substances for killing bacteria is boiling water.

---

## Tearing Down Mineral Buildup

So you've tried these formulas, but you're still having problems getting your bathroom surfaces adequately clean. Before you give up, remember that you may live in a hard water area. Hard water contains lots of minerals, and as you might have discovered from bitter experience, a portion of these minerals will stay behind on surfaces and accumulate. What's worse, these deposits create a rougher texture that more readily hold soap scum. But this hard-water buildup is not indestructible—nor will it require something as impractical as dynamite to remove.

You need acidic substances in order to eat into these mineral deposits. Lemon juice and vinegar possess this property. So the first thing to do is to try increasing their proportions in your cleaning formula.

If you require more abrasion, mix 1/4 cup of either of the ingredients with 1 teaspoon of alum. Use a bowl to combine, then take a rag, soak it well in the mixture, and rub on the buildup until it disappears. Rinse thoroughly. Repeat as many times as necessary.

---

## Suggested Mineral Deposit Cleaner

- 1/4 cup lemon juice or vinegar
- 1 teaspoon alum

❶ Place lemon juice or vinegar and alum in a bowl and mix
❷ Thoroughly soak rag in the mixture
❸ Rub on the accumulation
❹ Rinse well
❺ Repeat as many times as necessary

---

## Keeping Your Efforts from Going Down the Drain

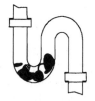

It usually happens when you are at your busiest and shortest on funds. There you are brushing your teeth, and you realize you're creating a small pond in your sink.

Don't panic. You might at least be able to avoid the plumber and save your money without resorting to the hard stuff (or a plunger). Wait for the water to drain. If the pipe is completely clogged, bail out as much water as you can and pour 1/2 cup of baking soda down the drain, then use 1/2 cup of lemon juice or vinegar as a chaser. You should hear it at work. Cover, let stand 15 minutes, and rinse with hot water.

---

## Suggested Drain Cleaner 1

- 1/2 cup baking soda
- 1/2 cup lemon juice or vinegar

❶ Pour baking soda down the drain
❷ Follow with lemon juice or vinegar
❸ Cover
❹ Let stand 15 minutes
❺ Rinse with hot water

---

A half cup of salt can be substituted for the vinegar or lemon juice. But if you use this method, follow up with 6 cups of boiling water. Allow it to sit at least several hours. Overnight would be better. Then flush with tap water.

---

## Suggested Drain Cleaner 2

- 1/2 cup baking soda
- 1/2 cup salt
- 6 cups boiling water

❶ Pour baking soda down the drain
❷ Follow with salt
❸ Add boiling water
❹ Cover
❺ Allow to sit several hours or overnight
❻ Then flush with tap water

---

To avoid such incidents in the future, there are several things that can be done. Most importantly, keep grease and large particles out of your sink (in the bathroom or kitchen). As an extra precaution, pour boiling water down the drains once or twice a week. If you want to go a step farther, add 1/2 cup of baking soda to 3 cups of boiling water and pour. Or pour 1/4 cup of washing soda down the drain and rinse with hot water.

So cleaning up the bathroom is really not so difficult after all. A few simple preventative measures and some basic cleaning formulas will make great strides toward washing away the dirt and mildew, not to mention your latest case of the "bathroom blues." In fact, once you become aware of just how effective these basic formulas really are, these cleaning chores almost might be considered fun.

# Chapter 2

# CARING FOR THE KITCHEN

## General Kitchen Cleaning

Here is an important point to remember about the kitchen when cleaning: Think high. Give a sufficient amount of time to dusting in the higher elevations. Cooking vapors move in that direction and quickly turn the dust that has deposited itself on appliances into a greasy film. For this reason, the hood of your range should be examined first. Regular cleaning, of course, is preferable to allowing this dusty buildup to develop.

Here are some suggested formulas for shining up your appliances. To a spray bottle, add 1 teaspoon of borax, 1/2 teaspoon of vegetable-oil-based liquid soap (optional), 3 tablespoons of vinegar, and 2 cups of hot water, then shake well. Apply to dirty surfaces and wipe dry with a sponge or soft cloth.

---

**Suggested Appliance Exterior Cleaner 1**

• 1 teaspoon of borax
• 3 tablespoons of vinegar
• 1/2 teaspoon of vegetable-oil-based liquid soap (optional)
• 1/2 teaspoon washing soda (optional)
• 2 cups of hot water

❶ Add ingredients to a spray bottle
❷ Shake well
❸ Apply to dirty surfaces with a rag or soft white nylon scrub brush
❹ Wipe dry with a sponge or soft cloth

---

When time is more important and the job is light, there is a quicker recipe. Just use 1/2 teaspoon of vegetable-oil-based liquid soap with 2 cups of water.

---

**Suggested Appliance Exterior Cleaner 2**

• 1/2 teaspoon of vegetable-oil-based liquid soap
• 2 cups of water

❶ Add ingredients to a spray bottle
❷ Shake well
❸ Apply to dirty surfaces with a rag or soft white nylon scrub brush
❹ Wipe dry with a sponge or soft cloth

---

If grease is an especially bad problem, add 1/2 teaspoon of washing soda to the above formula. Or, rub splatters with the inside of a citrus peeling.

---

**Suggested Appliance Exterior Cleaner 3**

• Citrus peeling

❶ Rub splatters with the inside of a citrus peeling
❷ Rinse with a soft moist cloth
❸ Dry with a clean cloth

---

And just as in the bathroom, mineral buildup can sometimes be a problem. The same formula can be used here as outlined in chapter 1. Another variation is to use a spray bottle containing 1 tablespoon of alum, 3 tablespoons of lemon juice or vinegar, and 2 cups of hot water.

---

**Suggested Appliance Exterior Cleaner 4**

• 1 tablespoon of alum
• 3 tablespoons of lemon juice or vinegar
• 2 cups of hot water

❶ Mix ingredients in a spray bottle
❷ Shake well
❸ Apply to dirty surfaces with a rag or soft white nylon scrub brush
❹ Wipe dry with a sponge or soft cloth

---

⊠ **Caution:** Since many appliances have a baked enamel surface, don't use steel wool or abrasive nylon scouring pads. They can cause damage. (A soft white nylon scrub brush is soft enough to be safe.)

---

❊ **Handy hint:** Use the scrub brush to apply your cleaner and a cloth to dry the surface.

❊ **Handy hint:** If you want your appliance surfaces especially shiny, use a glass cleaner to polish it. (See Chapter 7 for information on cleaning glass.)

Appliances have plastic and oil coatings on them when new. They will gradually burn off with the heat emitted during their use, but you can hasten the process by removing some of it ahead of time. For this job, use approximately 1 teaspoon of washing soda with 2 cups of hot water. Place in a spray bottle and apply to surfaces. Let it remain for at least an hour before rinsing.

❊ **Handy hint:** Your appliance knobs should be washed too because the serrated or grooved portions accumulate a lot of dirt. Often they slip off with little effort, but sometimes this requires the loosening of a small screw. Getting them off makes them easier to clean, in addition to the spots *under* the knob.

Also, vacuum the areas around your appliances at least once a month—especially the refrigerator. The grill at the bottom (kick plate) and coils in the rear can become encrusted with dust and affect the device's efficiency.

Kitchen counters, tables, cutting boards, electric can openers and similar surfaces can be cleaned with the same formulas suggested for your appliances. Cutting boards, especially, should be cleaned after each use to keep down the spread of bacteria. Just apply your favorite formula and rinse. And don't worry about it if you happen to spill club soda on a cabinet. It, too, is an effective cleaner. All you need to do is sponge it up and rinse.

---

**Suggested General Kitchen Cleaner**

• Club soda

❶ Apply with a sponge
❷ Rinse

---

## The Appliance Within

The outside surfaces, of course, are not the only part of appliances that must be cleaned. Don't forget about the *inside* surfaces too, as well as removeable items such as drawers, grills, covers, burner pans, and drip trays. The drip tray at the bottom of the refrigerator is especially important. It's another spot in the home where mildew can easily grow because of the high concentration of moisture. When cleaning this item, make certain you include borax in your formula to slow down the growth of the mildew. The recommended time for cleaning this item is once a month.

In addition, don't forget about the crumb tray of your toaster or toaster oven. When they are clean, it will prevent smoldering of leftover particles that can affect thermostats and sometimes make door-opening mechanisms difficult to operate.

As far the interior surfaces, the automatic dishwasher pretty well takes care of itself, although it might require an occasional damp cloth in the event there is stuck-on food or detergent debris. While you're looking, it wouldn't hurt to check the drain for any remains that may have lodged there.

The washing machine interior is also a low-maintenance surface. But once or twice a year, run your washer through a full cycle after filling it with warm water and several cups of vinegar. This will prevent future clogs by breaking up any soap scum that may be occupying the inside of the hoses.

---

### Suggested Washing Machine Interior Cleaner

- 2 or 3 cups of vinegar
- 1 load of warm water

❶ Fill washing machine with warm water
❷ Add vinegar
❸ Run through a full wash cycle

---

The refrigerator interior, meanwhile, can be handled with a baking soda and/or borax and warm water solution. Use approximately 2 tablespoons of soda or borax per quart of water. Straight vinegar can also be used. Be sure and keep the gasket along the inside of the door clean too. If enough dirt is allowed to buildup around it, some of the cool air will leak through it and reduce the efficiency of the appliance.

---

### Suggested Refrigerator Interior Cleaner 1

- 2 tablespoons baking soda or borax
- 1 quart warm water

❶ Mix ingredients
❷ Rub onto surfaces
❸ Rinse
❹ Dry

**Suggested Refrigerator Interior Cleaner 2**

• Vinegar

❶ Apply vinegar straight
❷ Rinse
❸ Dry

This same principle applies to microwave ovens. If the door seal is not tight, dangerous microwave radiation can leak out.

## The Search for Oven Heaven

But what about the kitchen range? There is nothing worse than facing the inside of a typical oven. No, this section offers no miracle cleaning solution, but the hardship it imposes does not have to be nearly as bad as you think. And it doesn't require toxic commercial oven cleaners, which are said to be one of the worst indoor air pollutants.

Believe it or not, baking soda or borax can be made to work just as well for this application. The key here is to strike while the iron is hot, so to speak, and do the cleaning while the surface is still slightly warm. If food residues prove particularly stubborn, add a little lemon juice. You can also use washing soda, but although it does well at cutting grease, it requires a more thorough rinsing. Still another idea is to sprinkle ordinary salt on oven spills before they have completely cooled.

## Suggested  Oven Cleaner  1

• Baking soda, borax, washing soda, or salt
• Lemon juice (optional)

❶ Sprinkle on any of these ingredients while the surface is still slightly warm
❷ Add lemon juice if stains are particularly stubborn
❸ Scrub with a mildly abrasive cleaning pad
❹ Rinse

## Suggested  Oven Cleaner  2

• Baking soda
• Water

❶ Sprinkle water over surface
❷ cover dried burned-on spills with baking soda
❸ Sprinkle more water over the soda
❹ Allow it to sit overnight

## Suggested  Oven Cleaner  3

• Salt
• Hot water

❶ Mix ingredients and apply to dried burned-on spills
❷ Allow to sit for a couple of hours or more
❸ Scrub
❹ Rinse

## Suggested Oven Cleaner 4

• Pumice bar

❶ Scrub stubborn burned-on spots
❷ Rinse

If you have waited too late and the oven is cold, sprinkle some water over the bottom surface, then cover the dried burned-on spills with baking soda. Distribute more water over the soda and allow it to sit overnight. Or add hot water and salt, and let it sit for at least a couple of hours.

## Suggested Oven Cleaner 5

• Baking soda
• Water

❶ Sprinkle water over surface
❷ cover dried burned-on spills with baking soda
❸ Sprinkle more water over the soda
❹ Allow it to sit overnight

## Suggested Oven Cleaner 6

• Salt
• Hot water

❶ Mix ingredients and apply to dried burned-on spills
❷ Allow to sit for a couple of hours or more
❸ Scrub
❹ Rinse

For best results, use a mildly abrasive cleaning pad (or a bar of pumice) to perform the job, then rinse. Better yet, prevent spills in the first place. Use adequate-sized containers, as well as a cookie sheet or a piece of aluminum foil beneath the cooking food in the event there is an overflow. Also, keep the dishes covered unless the recipe states otherwise. If using a microwave oven, stick to large ceramic or glass dishes that are microwave safe.

---

⊠ Caution: Try to keep your microwave at the 3 to 3 1/2 foot level. If it has been placed too high, the chances of spilling something out on top of yourself increases.

---

If something does happen to spill on your oven while you are in the process of cooking, try this quick fix. Quickly sprinkle the soiled area with table salt. It will mix with the material and the whole mess will be easier to scrape up after the oven has cooled down.

And while on the subject, also be sure to clean spoiled foods on top of your stove as soon as possible after cooking. It's a good idea, too, to go over the burners when they have cooled down enough. To minimize the need for such cleaning, adopt the habit of cooking more slowly. This will reduce the change of boil-overs. Or just as with the oven, you can cover the areas around your burners with sheets of aluminum foil. Then rather than having to scrub them when food is spilled or boils over, just replace the foil.

---

❊ **Handy hint:** Be sure to rinse any cleaning pads in hot water after use. Otherwise, grease and grime will harden in them.

---

⊠ **Caution:** If you own a self-cleaning oven, remember that it contributes to indoor pollution during the cleaning cycle. Make certain you have adequate ventilation.

---

## Overcoming Dish Drudgery

The time to clean dishes is directly after the meal—not later that night, or worse, the next morning. It's a temptation to do so, but if you put off this task, you'll be asking for a more difficult job. The food will have hardened, necessitating the use of more cleaning supplies and longer periods of scrubbing. And not only are soiled dishes unhealthy when allowed to sit, but they encourage the growth of bacteria. This, in turn, produces unpleasant odors and draws pests.

A vegetable-oil-based soap can be used with good results. For the scrubbing part of the job, use a cotton sponge or a dishwashing brush with replaceable heads.

---

**Suggested Dishwashing Cleaner 1**

• Vegetable-oil-based soap

❶ Apply soap to dish water
❷ Scrub with a cotton sponge or a dishwashing
brush with a replaceable head

---

If you prefer, you can make a mild dishwashing soap ahead of time. Soften a bar of unscented hand or bath soap by allowing it to soak in a jar of water for several days. Then smooth it in a blender. Or, for a faster and easier version, grate a bar of unscented soap into a pan. Make the gratings as small as you can to promote dissolving. Then cover with water and simmer over a low heat until melted. This process may require a couple of hours. Pour into a squeeze container and have at it.

---

**Suggested Homemade Dishwashing Soap 1**

• Homemade dishwashing soap

❶ Soften a bar of unscented hand or bath soap by
allowing to soak in a jar of water for several
days
❷ Then smooth in a blender
❸ Pour into squeeze container and use when
needed

---

## Suggested Homemade Dishwashing Soap 2

❶ Grate (as finely as possible) a bar of unscented soap into a pan
❷ Cover with water
❸ Simmer over a low heat until melted (perhaps as much as 2 hours)
❹ Pour into squeeze container and use when needed

❋ **Handy hint:** For tougher jobs, add 2 tablespoons of vinegar or lemon juice to your dish water, or 2 teaspoons of borax to the rinse water.

## Suggested Dishwashing Cleaner 2

• Vegetable-oil-based soap
• 2 tablespoons vinegar or lemon juice
• 2 teaspoons of borax

❶ Apply soap to dish water
❷ Then add vinegar or lemon juice for tougher jobs
❸ Or add borax to the rinse water

For stubborn buildup on pots and pans, avoid metal scrapers. Instead, soak them for awhile in a sink full of hot salty water. Then wash. Also, you can substitute washing soda or baking soda for the salt. (To learn more about how to clean specific metals, see Chapter 6.)

## Suggested Dishwashing Cleaner 3

• Salt, Washing Soda or baking soda
• Hot water

❶ Add salt, washing soda or baking soda to hot dish water
❷ Soak pots and pans with stubborn buildup
❸ Wash as usual

⊠ **Caution:** It is not recommended that you use washing soda, baking soda, or borax on aluminum on a continued basis. These substances will subject this metal to discoloration and eventual deterioration.

To clean coffeemakers (non-aluminum only), fill to the top with water and add 1 teaspoon of borax per cup. Allow the coffee maker to go through an entire brewing cycle, then wait 20 minutes and rinse well. Tea kettles can be handled the same basic way. Just add the ingredients and boil for at least 10 minutes. For aluminum, use 2 tablespoons of vinegar per cup of water instead of borax.

## Suggested Non-aluminum Coffeemaker Cleaner

• Water
• 1 teaspoon borax per cup of water

❶ Completely fill with water
❷ Add borax
❸ Complete an entire brewing cycle
❹ Wait 20 minutes
❺ Rinse well

## Suggested Non-Aluminum Tea Kettle Cleaner

• Water
• 1 teaspoon borax per cup of water

❶ Completely fill with water
❷ Add borax
❸ Boil for 10 minutes
❹ Rinse well

Note: For aluminum coffee makers and tea kettles, use 2 tablespoons of vinegar per cup of water instead of borax.

If you are plagued by cups with coffee or tea stains, rub with a salt/vinegar paste. While you're at it, you may as well mix up the paste with one of the stained cups.

## Suggested Dishwashing Cleaner 3

• Vinegar
• Salt

❶ Combine ingredients to make a paste
❷ Rub into cups with coffee or tea stains

For cleaning non-stick cookware (usually teflon), the rules change slightly. Place 3 tablespoons of baking soda and 3 lemon slices in the soiled teflon pot or pan and add enough water to cover the stains. Simmer on a flame until the stains have lifted. Then rinse thoroughly.

---

**Suggested Non-stick Cookware Cleaner**

• 3 tablespoons baking soda
• 3 lemon slices
• Water

❶ Place baking soda and lemon slices in the soiled pot or pan
❷ Add enough water to cover the stains
❸ Simmer on stove until stains have lifted
❹ Rinse thoroughly

---

Now all that's left is to dry what has been washed. You can do one of three things: reach for the dish rag, yell for volunteers or forget the whole thing. The best bet is to forget the whole thing. No kidding! Let them drip-dry in the dish drainer. It is more hygienic.

All right, so you're lucky. You have an automatic dishwasher (and no dishpan hands). You won't have to worry about drying, only eliminating the worst of the food buildup before you load to avoid the prospect of any residue getting lodged in the drain.

Unfortunately, there isn't much in the way of environmentally friendly substances that are completely effective in the dishwasher (although a teaspoon of borax is an excellent detergent supplement). So if you think you are physically affected by strong dishwashing detergents, it may be better to do those dishes by hand and use gentler cleaners. You can still make do with substituting borax for dishwashing detergent, however. Just use 1/4 cup for each washing cycle.

## Suggested Automatic Dishwashing Cleaner 1

• Borax

❶ Scrape away worst of food buildup on dishes before loading
❷ Add 1/4 cup borax instead of regular dishwashing detergent
❸ Or add 1 teaspoon of borax along with your detergent as a supplement

## Suggested Automatic Dishwashing Cleaner 2

• 2 cups vinegar

❶ Put dishes that have accumulated chalky de posits back in dishwasher
❷ Place a cup filled with vinegar on the bottom rack
❸ Let machine run for 5 minutes
❹ Then stop it
❺ Empty cup (which will now be filled with water)
❻ Refill with vinegar and place back in dish washer
❼ Complete cycle
❽ Rewash with dishwasher detergent if necessary

✽ **Handy hint:** It is not a good idea to store dishwasher detergent directly under the kitchen sink. Because of the amount of moisture present there, it can become easily caked. If it does, it may not completely dissolve and leave a residue on dishes.

If you do use the dishwasher, keep these facts in mind:

■ Dishwahers are not designed to wash heat-sensitive plastics and woodenware (this includes pots and pans with wooden handles), colored or high-gloss aluminumware, insulated glasses and cups, lacquered metal, ironware or delicate china.

■ Bacteria-free dishes are not guaranteed from using any dishwasher.

■ Smaller loads are more likely to get clean.

■ Even though there is an ingredient in some dishwasher detergents that is suppose to prevent spotting, there is no guarantee that spotting will not occur. Conditions such as water type, dishwasher brand and the amount of the load vary from home to home.

■ Spotting does not necessarily mean dishes are not clean.

■ An excessive amount of detergent can keep dishes from being cleaned effectively. It fills the water with too many suds and sometimes deposits a chalky residue on your kitchenware. (Keep in mind that soft water produces more suds.)

■ A temperature between 140° and 160° is recommended for efficient drying.

To remove chalky deposits left on dishes, place them back in the dishwasher and put a cup filled with vinegar on the bottom rack. Let the machine run for 5 minutes, then stop it. Empty the cup (which will now be filled with water) and refill it with vinegar, placing it back in the dishwasher. Complete the cycle. You may also have to rewash with dishwasher detergent.

---

### Suggested Automatic Dishwashing Cleaner 3

• 2 cups vinegar

❶ Put dishes that have accumulated chalky deposits back in dishwasher
❷ Place a cup filled with vinegar on the bottom rack
❸ Let machine run for 5 minutes
❹ Then stop it
❺ Empty cup (which will now be filled with water)
❻ Refill with vinegar and place back in dish washer
❼ Complete cycle
❽ Rewash with dishwasher detergent if necessary

---

## Disposing of Garbage and its Odors

Don't forget the garbage disposal. An excellent deodorizer for this device comes in the form of citrus. It doesn't necessarily have to be lemons—limes, grapefruits and oranges also work well. Simply drop some slices of any of these fruits into the disposal, including the rind, and grind. Then rinse with hot water.

For purposes of cleaning and disinfecting, pour 1/4 of a cup of borax or baking soda down the disposal (and other drains) every couple of weeks or so.

And here's an additional idea for keeping down odor. Every time you add a significant amount of trash to your garbage pail, sprinkle a little baking soda in it. This will also work, of course, for outside trash containers, particularly during the warmer seasons.

---

## Garbage Disposal Deodorizer 1

• Citrus (lemon, lime, orange, etc.)
• Hot water

❶ Drop some slices of any of these fruits, including the rind, into the disposal
❷ Grind
❸ Rinse with hot water

---

## Garbage Disposal Deodorizer 2

• 1/4 of a cup of borax or baking soda

● Pour borax or baking soda down the disposal (and other drains) every couple of weeks or so.

Note: Sprinkle a little baking soda in with your garbage pail to deodorize it.

---

So there you have it—the safest, most effective ways to clean your kitchen appliances and wash your dishes. Granted, it is not a totally painless job, but with a few simple ingredients and a little time, you will be able to keep your kitchen in top shape.

# Chapter 3

# COMING OUT IN THE WASH

## Washing Your Loads of Laundry

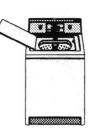

Whether in the kitchen, utility room, or even the garage, washing the clothes is as much a regular feature as the Sunday funnies. Unless there are stubborn stains to contend with, one of the best cleaning substances for this purpose is borax. It not only cleans, but also deodorizes, disinfects, whitens and acts as a water softener. If more abrasiveness is required, try adding table salt to the load. Salt will also prevent colors from running.

---

**Suggested General Clothes Washing Formula 1**

• Borax
• Salt (optional)

❶ Add to wash as you would a detergent
❷ Include table salt in the load for tougher jobs and to prevent colors from running

---

❋ **Handy hint:** The cabinet directly under the kitchen sink is a poor place to store borax and other powdered cleaners. Due to the amount of moisture present, these substances can become easily caked.

You can also make your own laundry soap. Just use the same process as that used for dishwashing soap. (See chapter 2). For a particularly good mixture, add borax to the soap to soften the water and washing soda to cut grease. Use hot water.

---

**Suggested General Clothes Washing Formula 2**

• Homemade laundry soap
• Borax (optional)
• Washing soda (optional)

❶ Make laundry soap the same way you make dishwashing soap
❷ Add to washer load
❸ Include borax if you require a water softener
❹ Include washing soda if there are a lot of greasy stains
❺ Use hot water

---

Another option is to buy perfume-free soap flakes. It is easier than making your own soap, but you'll have to shop around, because they're hard to find.

---

**Suggested General Clothes Washing Formula 3**

• Perfume-free soap flakes

❶ Add to load instead of homemade soap
❷ Include optional ingredients if desired

---

For natural fibers such as silk or wool, place 1 or 2 teaspoons of vegetable-oil-based liquid soap in the sink and add cold water. Mix until sudsy. Put garments in and cover with more water. Gently hand wash, then rinse thoroughly. If you feel you must use your washing machine for these kind of fabrics, make sure your agitation and spin speeds are set on low.

---

## Suggested Clothes Washing Formula 4

❶ For natural fibers such as silk or wool, place vegetable-oil-based liquid soap in sink
❷ Add cold water
❸ Mix until sudsy
❹ Put garments in and cover with more water
❺ Gently hand wash
❻ Rinse thoroughly

---

## Suggested Clothes Washing Formula 5

❶ Place soap and garments to your washing machine
❷ Wash on lowest speed

• 1/4 cup baking soda
• 1/8 cup vinegar
• 1/8 cup borax

---

❈ **Handy hint:** To avoid a grayish appearance in your clothes because of hard water (or sometimes due to excess soap), add 1/4 cup of baking soda, or 1/8 cup of vinegar or borax to the rinse cycle. If this gray color has been allowed to build up, it may require several washings to correct. Vinegar is also a help in that it reduces lint and static cling.

## The Best Ways to Bleach

For those who are particularly interested in bleaching, there are a few other procedures you can follow. For white clothing, add 2 or 3 tablespoons of sodium percarbonate to the load. (Check health food stores for sodium percarbonate.) Lemon juice, vinegar and washing soda can also be effective as a general bleach in addition to borax. Try adding 1/4 cup of any of these to the wash cycle whether you use soap.

---

## Suggested Bleaching Formula 1

• 2 or 3 tablespoons sodium percarbonate

● Add to your load of white clothing

---

## Suggested Bleaching Formula 2

• Borax
• Lemon juice
• Vinegar
• Washing soda

● Add 1/4 cup of any of the above ingredients to the wash cycle whether or not you use soap

---

Another option is to use the most basic ingredient of all. Forget the dryer and hang your clothes in the sun. Don't scoff—sunlight happens to be a natural bleach (as well as a disinfectant).

If you are bleaching individual articles, try this. Dissolve 1 tablespoon of borax in a quart of boiling water. Then pour in 1 quart of cold water. Dip in the soiled garment(s) and let dry in the sun. Repeat as many times as necessary.

## Suggested Bleaching Formula 3

- 1 tablespoon borax
- 1 quart boiling water
- 1 quart cold water
- Sunlight

❶ If you are bleaching individual articles, dissolve borax in boiling water
❷ Then pour in 1 quart of cold water
❸ Dip in soiled garment(s)
❹ Allow to dry in sun
❺ Repeat as many times as necessary

## Some Firm Advice About Starching

For starching jobs, all you need is cornstarch. Add several teaspoons of cornstarch and 2 cups of water to a spray bottle and shake well. Use as you would with any starch product. If you are starching dark garments, you can include 1/2 cup of black tea in the formula. Rinse the nozzle after each use to prevent it from becoming clogged. If you desire a scent with this formula, add a few drops of lemon juice.

---

## Suggested Starch Formula

- Several teaspoons cornstarch
- 2 cups water
- 1/2 cup black tea (optional)
- A few drops of lemon juice (optional)

❶ Add cornstarch and water to spray bottle
❷ Include tea if starching dark garments
❸ Include lemon juice if scent is desired
❹ Shake well
❺ Use as you would with any starch product
❻ Rinse nozzle after each use

---

## Those Stubborn Stains

Actually, washing clothes wouldn't be so bad if that was all there was to it. But what about perspiration marks or tough food stains? These annoying blemishes don't always disappear like magic.

The best bet is to perform the initial step of soaking the soiled garment(s). This will help soften the substance(s) that have already been set in the material. If the stain is still fresh, the first step is to blot, not rub it, with a clean white cloth and then treat. As a general rule, don't soak in hot water because it will set most stains.

Many of the same basic washing ingredients can be used—they just need to be applied directly to the spots as soon as possible. A good bet is to make a paste by adding small amounts of washing soda or baking soda to water. Then rub onto the areas preferably with an old toothbrush and allow to dry. Follow up with a machine wash.

❋ **Handy hint:** Use your brush on the stain before you add any cleaner, but don't rub in the conventional sense. This only serves to grind the unwanted matter deeper into the fabric and, in some cases, damage that fabric. And quite often it winds up expanding the stain. Instead, apply a gentle lifting motion and, depending on the type of stain, you may be able to knock some of the particles loose.

❋ **Handy hint:** Baking soda works well for removing perspiration stains, as does soaking the article in warm water and vinegar.

⊠ **Caution:** Baking soda is not recommended for wool.

Cream of tartar is another ingredient that can be used for stains. Follow the same procedure as with washing or baking soda. For stains on white articles, try making a paste with sodium perborate (if not available at your drug store, see "Chemical Supply Companies" in the yellow pages) or sodium percarbonate.

---

## Suggested Stain Remover 1

- Washing soda
- Baking soda
- Cream of tartar
- Water

❶ Make a paste by adding small amounts of washing soda, baking soda or cream of tartar to water
❷ Rub onto the areas with an old toothbrush
❸ Allow to dry
❹ Follow up with a machine wash

---

## Suggested Stain Remover 2

- Sodium perborate or sodium percarbonate Water

❶ For stains on white articles, make a paste with sodium perborate or sodium percarbonate and water
❷ Apply to stain
❸ Allow to dry
❹ Follow up with machine wash

---

Salt and vinegar are also effective for removing perspiration stains. Place soiled clothes in the washing machine. Add 1/4 cup of either to the soiled clothes and fill with just enough water to cover them. Then agitate and allow to sit overnight before washing.

Also, many kinds of stains can be removed with this general cleaner: 1 part vegetable glycerin (found at pharmacies or health food stores), 1 part vegetable-oil-based liquid soap and 8 parts water.

---

**Suggested Stain Remover 3**

- 1 part vegetable glycerin
- 1 part vegetable-oil-based liquid soap
- 8 parts water

❶ Mix ingredients
❷ Apply to stain
❸ Wash as usual

---

For tough stains on linen or cotton clothing, apply lemon juice, then sprinkle with salt and allow to dry in the sun.

---

**Suggested Stain Remover 4**

- Lemon juice
- Salt
- Sunlight

❶ For tough stains on linen or cotton clothing, apply lemon juice
❷ Sprinkle with salt
❸ Allow to dry in the sun

---

You can also consider the use of hair shampoo for stain removal. Just rub some into the dirty area and wash. (Look in health food stores for shampoos, as they will tend to contain ingredients that are more environmentally friendly.)

---

**Suggested  Stain Remover 5**

• Hair shampoo

❶ Rub into stain
❷ Wash as usual

---

For rings around collars and cuffs, it is often helpful to rub them heavily with a stick of white chalk and allow them to sit awhile before washing. This will absorb the body oil which attracted the dirt in the first place.

---

**Suggested Stain Remover  6**

• Stick of white chalk

❶ Heavily rub rings around collars and cuffs with chalk
❷ Allow garment(s) to sit awhile
❸ Wash

---

For diapers, put 1/4 to 1/2 cup of borax in a diaper pail of hot water. Presoak for a while, then wash. Flush out heavily soiled diapers before soaking.

---

**Suggested Diaper Cleaner**

- 1/4 to 1/2 cup of borax
- Diaper pail of hot water

❶ For diapers, fill pail with hot water
❷ Mix in borax
❸ Add diapers (flushing out those that are heavily soiled first)
❹ Presoak for awhile
❺ Then wash

---

So you have some stains that are extra stubborn. Admittedly, there are many: chocolate, fruit juices, blood, grass, rust, to name a few—and most of them, unfortunately, must be handled differently. But don't fret. There are still other simple products that can be put to use for these specific purposes:

■ Remove **alcoholic beverage** stains by using vinegar or alcohol. If this fails, try bleaching carefully with hydrogen peroxide. Dilute these cleaners with at least 2 parts of water when applying to delicate fabrics. These procedures are also effective for **perfume**.

■ Wash **antiperspirant** stains with warm water and vegetable-oil-based soap. If they prevail after rinsing, try applying vinegar, hydrogen peroxide or sodium perborate and rinse again.

■ **Baby formula** stains can be rubbed with meat tenderizer (unseasoned).

■ Wipe **blood** stains with hydrogen peroxide, make a paste from cornstarch or cornmeal and rub into the spot, or rinse with club soda. You can also try soaking in salt water for several hours. In addition, blood stains can be rubbed with unseasoned meat tenderizer and left on the soiled area for at least a half hour. Yet another method is to rub aggressively with an ice cube. Nothing more than clear, cold water can be effective if applied before the stain has had a chance to set.

■ For **chocolate** stains not removed by any of the general cleaning formulas, try wiping with hydrogen peroxide. Glycerin can also be of help. Sponging with cold water will keep this kind of stain from setting.

■ **Coffee** or **tea** spots that survive any of the general formulas may be more successful handled by increasing the quantity of vinegar used or allowing the article to soak in a strong vinegar/water solution. You can also rub these stains with vegetable glycerin before washing. Cold water will prevent coffee stains from setting; hot water will keep tea stains from setting.

■ Rub **crayon** marks and **lipstick** stains with toothpaste. Most of the crayon residue can also be removed by placing an absorbent cloth over it and ironing. This will melt the wax into the cloth. As a general rule, **cosmetic** stains can be removed with a vegetable-oil-based soap.

■ Use cold water when washing out **egg** stains. Scrape off as much as you can and then sponge or soak the article.

■ Try rinsing general **food** stains with club soda or vegetable-oil-based liquid soap and vinegar.

■ For **fruit** stains, try one of the following: Stretch fabric over the sink and pour boiling water through the stained area, rub with vegetable glycerin and allow to remain for approximately 1 hour before washing, or soak the soiled garment in milk or white wine. The same technique goes for **wine** stains. Do not launder in hot water as that will set the stain. If the stain is from a richer colored fruit, e. g. berry or grape, apply lemon juice, rinse, and blot out as much moisture as you can. Then allow to finish drying.

■ For mild **glue**, use a vegetable-oil-based liquid soap before it has dried. If it has already hardened, you may be able to remove it by soaking (non-delicate items only) in hot vinegar maintained at the boiling point for 15 minutes or more.

■ **Grass** smudges and other plant stains that escape the general cleaning formulas may have to be soaked in a solution of 1 part alcohol and 2 parts water. (Note: Substitute vinegar for alcohol if dealing with delicate fabrics such as silk, wool or acetate.) You can also try glycerin. Just rub into the stain and allow it to remain for at least 1 hour, then wash. Apply hydrogen peroxide or sodium perborate to any stains that persist.

■ Bread, wheat bran, cornstarch, cornmeal, kitty litter, chalk dust or talcum powder can be effective in removing **grease** spots. They serve as excellent absorbents. Apply and rinse several times if necessary, then wash in the conventional manner. If grease spots are completely dry, an absorbent will not do much good. The garment should be washed with a vegetable-oil-based soap, washing soda and borax.

■ If vinegar does not work in removing **gum** or **other sticky items**, freeze the area with ice cubes or place the garment in the freezer for a while. Then the gum should peel off easily. This approach will also work for removing **candle wax**. Wax can also be removed by applying blotting paper and pressing with a hot iron. The paper may have to be changed several times before all of the wax is absorbed.

■ **Ink** spots not removed by the general cleaning measures may need to be soaked in a solution of vinegar, cornstarch and milk. Alcohol and glycerin may also do the trick. If these procedures fail, treat them as you would rust stains. (Note: alcohol may cause some dyes to bleed.)

■ Rub **iodine** stains and **nail polish** with alcohol. If necessary, place a pad of alcohol-soaked cotton on the spot and keep it there for several hours. Since alcohol evaporates so quickly, you will have to remoistening the cotton periodically.

■ If the general formulas are not effective enough for **mildew**, rub the affected spots with Australian tea tree oil (available at health food stores). Drying in the sun after washing is also a great help.

■ For **milk** stains, rinse in cold water and wash. Soak delicate fabrics in 1 part glycerin and 1 part warm water, then rub gently until the stain loosens, and soak in alcohol for approximately 2 minutes. Follow by washing.

■ **Mud** stains not removed by normal washing can be eliminated with alcohol.

■ Try rubbing **mustard** stains with vegetable glycerin. If the stain still shows, use a bleach such as hydrogen peroxide or sodium perborate.

■ **Nail polish** can be removed with alcohol.

■ Spots of **oil** may need to be rubbed with vegetable or nut oil, or cornmeal or kitty litter.

■ If washing soda does not remove **paint**, soak in milk or hot vinegar.

■ For **perfume** stains, wash in warm water if fresh. Set stains should be rubbed with glycerin.

Allow glycerin to remain for at least 1 hour on nonwashables, then sponge with warm water. (See also **alcoholic beverage**.)

■ Alum or salt may have to be added to lemon juice or vinegar to remove **rust** stains. Another method is to rub rust spots with cooked, cooled rhubarb. Still another idea is to boil the soiled article in a solution containing 4 teaspoons of cream of tartar per pint of water.

■ If **shoe polish** can't be removed by the use of a vegetable-oil-based soap, try sponging it with alcohol.

■ **Smoke** or **soot** blemishes not remedied by the

use of an absorbent such as washing soda or borax may be removed with a vegetable-oil-based soap. You can also try hydrogen peroxide.

■ For **tar**, scrap of as much of it as possible and soak the affected article in cool water overnight. Then apply a vegetable-oil-based soap. If the stain still lingers, use hydrogen peroxide or sodium perborate.

■ Soak garments with **tobacco** stains in a mild vinegar solution, then wash. Repeat if necessary. Add baking soda to the formula to reduce smoke odor. Alcohol is also effective.

■ Most any of the general cleaning formulas will do for **urine**. Blot up as much as you can first, then apply the ingredients. (Note: Since urine is acidic, baking soda is excellent to include in your formula. It will neutralize the acid.)

■ Commercial **wood stains** that have soiled clothing can be dealt with by soaking in 1 part milk and 1 part vinegar before washing. An alternate formula involves the use of 1 part vegetable glycerin and 2 parts vegetable-oil-based liquid soap.

---

⊠ **Caution:** It is suggested that you test any of the above formulas on concealed or inconspicuous areas of clothing such as the underside of a collar or an unexposed seam before using it on a full scale basis, particularly those involving bleaches. In addition, these formulas should be diluted when used on fine fabrics or not used on them at all if you feel there is any possibility that they could be damaged.

---

⊠ **Caution:** Do not purchase too much hydrogen peroxide at one time. It eventually loses its strength.

---

❋ **Handy hint:** Try applying lemon juice to any stains that prove especially stubborn, and hang the garment in the sun. This does not mean you have to use a clothes line, either. If you spread out an old sheet on a table or even the ground and lay the article(s) on it, you will get the maximum benefit from the sun's rays.

---

There is no guarantee that every stain can automatically be removed. It depends on a number of factors such as the kind of material, its age, the exact ratio of ingredients you use, and water hardness. Sometimes it will require several applications before complete success can be achieved, in other in stances it will prove hopeless. Certainly in some cases, it would be less trouble to discard the garments, if not consign them for use when, for instance, you next decide to clean out the garage. If stains simply will not go away after countless washings, if you have owned the article for half your life, if it has begun to deteriorate anyway, or if the stain could more accurately be termed "damage," then it is time to give up and purchase new attire.

In summary, hand wash delicate garments or use the delicate setting on your washing machine. Observe all cautions mentioned above. Treat all stains as soon as possible; the longer you wait, the tougher the job will be because the stains will begin to set. Don't overdo the soap; too much in a load can leave a soap film on your clothes. And, of course, never overload your washing machine.

# Chapter 4

# FARING WELL WITH FURNITURE

## Being a Successful Dustbuster

Before discussing the cleaning formulas, let's touch on some basics concerning general dusting:

■ Always dust before you vacuum. You can imagine how disheartening it would be to discover that your dust rag was sending cookie crumbs off onto a freshly vacuumed carpet.

■ Aim high. Attack light fixtures, lofty shelves and door frames first. Then progress downward to tables, chairs, pianos, etc. That way you'll be saving all the fallout for the vacuum cleaner.

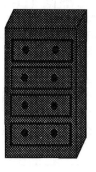

■ To maximize time, pick a day each week to give the most convenient areas a reasonable once-over. Shift your attention to less accessible areas such as door frames and light fixtures only on a monthly basis.

■ Forget feather dusters. They only serve to distribute dust into the air. Stick to appropriately moistened dust rags or particle-attracting dusters. (More on that shortly.)

Don't assume you have to make a ritual of polishing all of your wood surfaces every time you touch a dust rag to them. Oily exteriors can promote the very problem you are trying to avoid by *attracting* dust. Concentrate mostly on the dusting process itself.

There is nothing better than a soft, slightly moist terry cloth or cotton rag to do the job. You won't incur damages to surfaces unless you expose them to excessive dampness. Have several cloths standing by. Use one until it has become saturated with dust, then switch to another one. For glossy surfaces, follow up with a dry cloth.

Another idea is to use an electrostatic cloth. It is composed of a fabric that picks up and holds dirt. You will be able to use it for awhile, but it will become saturated. No problem, though. All you have to do is throw it in the washing machine and it'll be as good as new.

A third option is a lambswool duster. Nothing more than a ball of wool attached to a long handle, it resembles cotton candy on a stick. It works much like the electrostatic cloth to attract dust. When it gets dirty, it can be vacuumed. Because it has a long handle, it's especially convenient for reaching high places and avoiding stooping when cleaning low areas.

---

❋ **Handy hint:** Don't rub cobwebs into surfaces trying to clean them away. If you use a flicking motion, they should come off much easier. The best tool for this job is the lambswool duster.

---

## Polishing and Waxing Your Furniture

When you do want to enhance your work with a polish, there is nothing wrong with olive oil or vegetable oil combined with lemon juice or vinegar. Just mix up one of these solutions in a glass jar and use it whenever you are ready.

## Suggested Furniture Polish 1

- 2 parts olive oil or vegetable oil
- 1 part lemon juice or vinegar

❶ Combine either oil with lemon juice or vinegar in glass jar
❷ Seal jar
❸ Use when needed by buffing with a soft cloth

✽ **Handy hint:** The proportions you use will depend upon what you prefer. If you go heavier on the oil, you will achieve a heavier mixture, whereas adding more juices will render a lighter formula. Oils will enrich wood; vinegar and lemon juice will bring up the dust. Whatever ratio you decide upon, the formula should be applied in a thin coat.

⊠ **Caution:** Any pre-existing wax on furniture can be dissolved by the use of vinegar. If you desire to protect the wax, cut back on the amount of vinegar you use in your formula.

There are other good combinations as well. You can combine lemon juice, vinegar and linseed oil. Or walnut oil and lemon juice. Or almond oil and lemon juice. Or walnut oil and lemon oil. Or lemon juice, linseed oil and—yes—whiskey.

## Suggested Furniture Polish 2

- 1 part lemon juice
- 1 part vinegar
- 4 parts linseed oil

❶ Combine ingredients in glass jar
❷ Seal jar
❸ Use when needed by buffing with soft cloth

## Suggested Furniture Polish 3

- 2 parts walnut oil
- 1 part lemon juice

● Follow previous instructions

## Suggested Furniture Polish 4

- 2 parts almond oil
- 1 part lemon juice

● Follow previous instructions

## Suggested Furniture Polish 5

- Walnut oil
- Lemon oil

● Follow previous instructions

## Suggested Furniture Polish 6

- 1 part lemon juice
- 4 parts linseed oil
- 1 part whiskey

● Follow previous instructions

If you happen to own furniture with raw wood surfaces, they *must* be treated. Failure to do so will cause them to dry out and crack. The best preventative medicine for them is a straight oil treatment such as lemon, linseed or olive oil. Take your time when applying so the wood will have a chance to absorb it. Any excess should be wiped off.

⊠ **Caution:** Go easy on oils. They are very strong. And when purchasing them, read the label carefully. Some contain synthetic additives.

But dusting and polishing may not always be enough. There is nothing to match the sheen and protection that a good wax provides. For this purpose, beeswax and mineral oil come to the rescue. Place a double boiler on low heat and add these ingredients in the top half. Try for approximately 2 tablespoons of beeswax and 1/2 of a cup of the oil. Allow the wax to melt. Mix by stirring. Pour the still-hot contents into a wide-mouthed, heat resistant vessel and allow to cool. When the wax has solidified, cut it into sections and remove. To use it, simply apply some to your furniture surfaces, then rub in with a soft rag. Some vinegar on your cloth will help smooth the wax.

You don't have to be stuck with mineral oil if you don't want to. Use lemon oil, olive oil or any other oil of your choice. And feel free to experiment with the ratio. The more wax you include in the formula, the heavier the formula will be, but the harder it will be to apply.

---

## Suggested Furniture Waxes

- 2 tablespoons beeswax
- 1/2 cup mineral oil, olive oil or lemon oil
- Vinegar (optional)

❶ Place beeswax and one of above oils in top half of double boiler
❷ Turn on low heat
❸ Stir occasionally, allowing wax to melt
❹ Pour the still hot contents into wide-mouthed vessel
❺ Allow to cool
❻ When wax has solidified, cut into sections and remove
❼ Rub into furniture surfaces when needed with soft rag
❽ Add vinegar to rag if desired

---

## Answers to Your Special Wood Problems

So much for maintenance. But what about spills on an unprotected coffee table or scratches on a chest of drawers?

No reason to fret. Even the answers to these problems are within arm's reach. If you have a fireplace, mix some wood ashes with a tablespoon of vegetable oil until you have a paste. Then simply rub onto the water-stained area. For those without easy access to ashes, use a corn oil/salt paste.

## Suggested Wood Furniture Stain Formula 1

• Wood ashes
• 1 tablespoon vegetable oil

❶ Mix wood ashes with vegetable oil until you have a paste
❷ Lightly rub into affected area with soft cloth

## Suggested Wood Furniture Stain Formula 2

• 1 tablespoon corn oil
• Salt

● Follow above instructions

Still another formula to use for water spots is 2 cups of vodka combined with a dozen drops of lemon oil. Lightly rub this mixture into the affected area with a soft cloth. Dry immediately because if the alcohol is allowed to sit, it will dissolve varnished surfaces.

## Suggested Wood Furniture Stain Formula 3

• 2 cups of vodka
• 12 drops of lemon oil

❶ Mix ingredients
❷ Lightly rub into affected area with soft cloth
❸ Dry immediately

❋ **Handy hint:** Corn oil and salt or vodka and lemon oil are the best of the formulas. Although ashes are capable of removing stains, the carbon they contain can sometimes produce stains of their own.

Scratches can often be hidden with a simple pecan or walnut. Break one of these nuts in half to expose the inside of the meat, and brush it across the damaged area until it fades. You can also concoct a homemade wood stain by boiling the ground shells of these nuts in water. Sometimes, rubbing an extra amount of the oil you use for polishing into scratches will be sufficient.

## Suggested Scratch Formula 1

• Pecan or Walnut

❶ Break nut in half
❷ Brush broken end across damaged area until it fades

For furniture made from dark woods such as mahogany, try applying iodine. Then polish the entire surface with the formula of your choice. If the iodine is too dark, mix with vinegar and you will achieve a lighter color. Gradually add the iodine to a small amount of vinegar until you have the exact shade you need, then apply.

**Suggested Scratch Formula 2**

• Iodine
• Vinegar (optional)

❶ Apply iodine to furniture made from dark woods
❷ If necessary, add iodine to a small amount of vinegar until you have exact shade you need
❸ Then polish entire surface with formula of your choice

You can also take care of scorch marks. Obtain some steel wool (the finest grade available) and gently rub the affected area, making sure your motion follows the direction of the grain. Then clean away the remaining particles with a sponge saturated in vinegar or lemon juice.

**Suggested Scorch Mark Formula**

• Finest grade steel wool
• Vinegar or lemon juice

❶ Gently rub affected area, following the direction of the grain
❷ Then clean away the remaining particles with a sponge saturated in vinegar or lemon juice

Another solution for eliminating minor stains, including scorch marks, involves the use of rottenstone (available in paint stores). Dip a cloth in linseed oil, then in powdered rottenstone and apply. Cover only small areas at a time, and always follow the direction of the grain. Follow up by wiping the surface with another cloth dampened with pure linseed oil, then complete the job by polishing with a dry cloth. Pumice can be used instead of rottenstone.

This technique may even work for ink stains if they have not penetrated the wood.

---

**Suggested Minor Stain  Formula**

• Powdered rottenstone or pumice
• Linseed oil

❶ Dip a cloth in linseed oil
❷ Then dip in rottenstone or pumice
❸ Gently rub affected area, following the direction of the grain
❹ Follow up by wiping surface with another cloth dampened with pure linseed oil
❺ Then polish with a dry cloth

---

If paint is the culprit, and it has not yet dried, wash off as much as you can with vegetable-oil-based soap and water, then proceed to polish. For dried paint spots, apply linseed oil and allow it to remain for awhile. This will soften them enough so that they can be scraped away. But do it carefully and follow up by rubbing off any additional residue with a cloth that has been dampened with a rottenstone/linseed oil paste. Then finish up by wiping with pure linseed oil.

---

**Suggested Fresh Paint  Stain  Formula**

• Vegetable-oil-based soap
• Water

❶ Wash off as much as possible with vegetable-oil-based soap and water
❷ Then polish

---

---

## Suggested Dried Paint Stain Formula

• Linseed oil
• Powdered rottenstone

❶ Apply oil and allow to remain until spots have softened
❷ Then scrap carefully
❸ Follow up by rubbing off any additional residue with a cloth dampened with a rottenstone/lin seed oil paste
❹ Then wipe with pure linseed oil

---

But what if one of the children has "embellished" one of your furniture surfaces with decals? Nothing to fret over. Pour olive oil on them and let it sit for the night. The next morning, rub with a soft rag. Vinegar can be used instead of olive oil on painted furniture.

---

## Suggested Decal Remover Formula

• Olive oil or vinegar

❶ Pour oil on decals (or vinegar if painted furniture is involved)
❷ Allow to sit overnight
❸ The next morning, rub with a soft rag

---

## Uprooting Upholstery Dirt

All furniture, of course, is not made exclusively of wood. It often contains cushions and/or are fitted with padding that is covered with cloth, vinyl or leather. The same general formulas outlined earlier for cleaning clothes in Chapter 3 are effective for these surfaces, too.

For fabric upholstery, use the foam from a liquid soap and water solution. Try mixing a 1/8 cup of vegetable-oil-based soap with 1 or 2 tablespoons of water in a wide-mouthed container. Simply extract the foam that is formed on the surface and apply as needed. For leather, rub beaten egg whites into stains. Vinyl can be cleaned satisfactorily with vegetable-oil-based soap and water or a 50/50 solution of water and vinegar. You can also use vegetable-oil-based soap for leather, but never wax it. In each case, be sure to rinse thoroughly.

---

## Suggested Fabric Upholstery Cleaner

- 1/8 cup vegetable-oil-based-liquid soap
- 1 or 2 tablespoons of water

❶ Mix soap and water in a wide-mouthed container
❷ Extract foam that is formed on surface
❸ Apply as needed
❹ Rinse thoroughly

---

## Suggested Leather Upholstery Cleaner 1

- Beaten egg whites

❶ Rub into stains
❷ Rinse thoroughly

## Suggested Leather Upholstery Cleaner 2

- Vegetable-oil-based soap
- Water

❶ Mix and rub into stains
❷ Rinse thoroughly

## Suggested Leather Upholstery Cleaner 3

- Warm olive oil

❶ Rub with above oil to restore the resilience of old leather
❷ Finish by polishing with a clean soft cloth
❸ Repeat as often as necessary

## Suggested Vinyl Upholstery Cleaner 1

- Vegetable-oil-based soap
- Water

● Follow above instructions

## Suggested Vinyl Upholstery Cleaner 2

- 1 part vinegar
- 1 part water

● Follow above instructions

To restore the resilience of old leather, rub it with olive oil. Warm the oil and the material will absorb it more efficiently. Finish by polishing with a soft cloth. Repeat as often as necessary.

To put it simply, you don't need potent polishes and waxes with extra ingredients to keep your furniture clean. Your choice of natural oils and a few basic cleaners are all that is usually necessary for the job.

# Chapter 5

# NOW YOU HAVE THE FLOOR

## Working With Conventional Vacuuming Devices

No one can be reminded of floors without considering the vacuum cleaner. Most use the conventional upright kind or the rolling canister type. These are fine for picking up the bits of debris that are visible to the unaided eye and they do make the carpets *appear* cleaner. But finer dust particles escape the porous bag, mix with the air, and eventually land back on the carpet, as well as accumulate on furniture surfaces.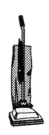

To minimize this problem, here are some tips to consider when replacing the bag in these devices:

■ Replace the bag when it's half full. Your machine is more efficient when it is operating with a lighter load.

■ Change the bag out-of-doors—always—even if you must wait for appropriate weather conditions. It's a messy job that will result in the escape of a certain amount of dust—and you don't want that dust to remain inside.

■ Clean the area around the bag with a moist cloth before installing a fresh bag. That will remove much of the excess dust.

■ Run the machine for at least 30 seconds before returning it to the house so any more loose dust that remains will be expelled.

There is another trick that will help the cause. Accessory filters are available that can be used with canister-type vacuum cleaners. When added, these filters reduce the number of particles emitted into the air.

If you decide to give this kind of filter a whirl, it must be changed regularly or its purpose will be defeated. If a blockage occurs out of neglect, debris can be forced through the sides of the filter, the mechanism could lose suction, or the motor could overheat. (See the yellow pages under "Vacuum Cleaners" for firms that furnish this type of filter.)

When you vacuum, do it as efficiently as possible. Try to maintain a consistent pattern. Begin at the fartherest corner of each room and work toward the doorway. It's best to keep the cord on the same side of you. If you're pressed for time, hit the areas that accommodate the heaviest amount of traffic.

---

❋ **Handy hint:** It would be a good idea to have your carpeting steam cleaned at least once a year. A lot of finer debris remains in your carpet that conventional vacuum cleaners don't have the ability to remove.

---

## Conquering Carpet Challenges

When you want to clean carpeting, keep in mind what each basic environmentally friendly ingredient best accomplishes. Baking soda, for instance, absorbs odors, while borax kills mold and vinegar eats away at stains.

If you want to eliminate pet odor, liberally sprinkle baking soda on your carpet and allow it to sit overnight. Vacuum the next day.

If, on the other hand, a section of your carpet has gotten wet, chances are mildew will begin growing there, and that means a shot of borax. After you sprinkle it around, it must be rubbed in with a cloth. It too should sit overnight before it is vacuumed.

In the event someone spills a drink, you'll do well to break out the vinegar.

Best yet, try these substances in combination to cover every possibility. Carpeting is typically affected by dirt, odor and mold alike.

---

## Suggested Carpet Cleaner 1

• Baking soda

❶ Sprinkle liberally on carpet to absorb pet odor
❷ Allow it to sit overnight
❸ Vacuum the next day

---

## Suggested Carpet Cleaner 2

• Borax

❶ Sprinkle on mildewed carpet
❷ Rub in with a cloth
❸ Allow to sit overnight
❹ Vacuum the next day

---

## Suggested Carpet Cleaner 3

• Vinegar or vodka

● Apply to minor spills

---

There are more interesting options. You might want to combine salt with the freshly cut side of a raw potato or the freshly cut side of a cabbage head and rub into dirty areas of your carpet. As the edges become dirty, re-cut, salt again, and continue to use. Of course, you will need to vacuum afterward. In each case, make sure the carpet is dry before application.

---

## Suggested Carpet Cleaner 4

• Salt
• Raw potato or cabbage head

❶ Salt freshly-cut side of potato or cabbage head
❷ Rub into dirty areas of (dry) carpet
❸ As edge becomes dirty, re-cut, salt again, and continue to use
❹ Vacuum afterward

---

For stains, however, you should attack them while they are still fresh. They will be much easier to remove then. Carefully blot up or pick up as much of the excess as you can, then apply the appropriate stain remover. (Check Chapter 3 for details.)

In addition, club soda is generally effective for carpet stains, too. Add a little salt with the club soda and you have a good coffee stain remover. Let the ingredients stand for a minute, then wipe up with a moist sponge. Salt, by the way, is useful for rubbing into mud spots. Let sit awhile and then vacuum. A carpet stain can also be rubbed with an alcohol such as vodka and rinsed with vinegar.

---

**Suggested Carpet Cleaner 5**

- Club soda
- Salt

❶ Pour on club soda
❷ Add a handful of salt
❸ Allow ingredients to stand a minute
❹ Then wipe up with a moist sponge

---

For specific problems such as cigarette burns, you may be able to remove singed fibers of carpeting, believe it or not, by scraping them with a silver coin. If soot is the plight, cover it with a thick layer of salt, then sweep. Do not wet it, however, as that will only make the stain worse.

To brighten carpet that has faded, vacuum, then dip a cloth in a 1 quart of vinegar and 3 gallons of boiling water solution and apply. (Use sparingly, because if the cloth becomes saturated, the liquid can penetrate the backing.) Next allow the carpet to thoroughly dry and rub with warm bread crumbs. Vacuum again.

---

## Suggested Carpet Cleaner 6

- 1 quart vinegar
- 3 gallons boiling water
- Warm bread crumbs

❶ Vacuum carpet
❷ Combine vinegar and water
❸ Then lightly dip cloth in solution and apply
❹ Next allow carpet to thoroughly dry
❺ Rub with warm bread crumbs
❻ Vacuum again

Note: For specific carpet stains, see Chapter 3.

---

✹ **Caution:** Never use salt water on carpeting. It can rot the backing.

---

## Making a Clean Sweep of It

Debris, of course, can also be vacuumed off of hard flooring. But often, you undoubtedly reach for the broom when it comes to small jobs. It beats lugging in the vacuum cleaner and its attachments. However, sweeping can stir up potential allergy-producing matter. In fact, a lot of particles remain on a broom—some to be released by air currents whenever the broom closet is opened. It would be far better to use a mop instead of a broom, even if it is only moistened with a few dabs of water.

If you do sweep, sprinkle some damp tea leaves around the floor first. This will keep the dust down. If the yard has just been mowed, snatch a handful of the freshly cut grass, and use that instead. Cornstarch also serves the same purpose. If nothing else, at least dampen the floor with a small amount of water from a spray bottle before sweeping. In addition, try wetting the inside of your dust pan.

## Floor Cleaning Made Easy

Floors need at least some measure of cleaner on a regular basis, whether it be wood, linoleum, terrazzo, vinyl or whatever. Again, the same basic ingredients used for other hard surface cleanups covered in chapters 1 and 2 can be employed for this purpose, too.

---

⊠ **Caution:** Although washing soda is acceptable for cleaning floors, keep in mind that it can dissolve wax. It is an excellent ingredient, however, to use as a wax *remover*, especially when combined with vinegar.

---

Try adding some herb tea to one of the formulas. A good combination would be 1/2 cup of lemon juice, a few tablespoons of vegetable-oil-based liquid soap, and 1/2 cup of the tea in 2 gallons of warm water. Just mix everything in a pail until sudsy and go for the mop.

---

### Suggested Hard Floor Cleaner 1

• 1/2 cup lemon juice
• A few tablespoons vegetable-oil-based liquid soap
• 1/2 cup herb tea
• 2 gallons of warm water

❶ Add ingredients to pail of warm water
❷ Mix until sudsy
❸ Mop as usual

Or combine 1/2 cup of lemon juice, a tablespoon of vegetable-oil-based liquid soap, and several drops of pennyroyal with a gallon of warm water. Then mop and rinse well. The pennyroyal serves as a flea repellant.

---

## Suggested Hard Floor Cleaner 2

- 1/2 cup lemon juice
- 1 tablespoon vegetable-oil-based liquid soap
- Several drops of pennyroyal
- 1 gallon warm water

❶ Combine lemon juice, soap and pennyroyal with warm water
❷ Mop
❸ Rinse well

---

⊠ **Caution:** The use of pennyroyal has been known to affect pregnant women. If you are pregnant or are planning to conceive, do not use pennyroyal.

---

For both spills and stains, alcohol will often work wonders. Just moisten a clean cloth with some, and rub. It doesn't necessarily have to be rubbing alcohol. Brandy or vodka can also be used.

---

## Suggested Hard Floor Cleaner 3

- Alcohol

❶ For stains, moisten clean cloth with alcohol
❷ Rub into stain

If you're plagued with tar, chill the area with ice cubes. This will make the tar brittle and it can be easily scraped up. But don't use a metal utensil when doing so, because it could mar your surface. A plastic spatula is a better choice.

---

**Suggested Tar Cleaner**

• Ice cubes

❶ To remove tar, chill area with ice cubes
❷ Scrap up with plastic spatula

---

✸ **Handy hint:** Try an ordinary eraser to take care of heel skid marks.

---

⊠ **Caution:** Do not use water on unfinished wood surfaces. It can raise the grain and eventually cause rot.

## Don't Let Waxing be Taxing

So you're interested in waxing your floors. (Even no-wax floors can eventually lose some of their luster.) Mixing an oil with beeswax will work for them just as with furniture. Again, you should experiment with proportions to achieve the consistency that best fits your needs.

---

✸ **Handy hint:** The best oil for the job is linseed oil. It dries quicker than other oils. And, of course, the faster a floor dries, the sooner it will be able to be walked on.

---

## Suggested Floor Wax

- Beeswax
- Linseed oil or other oil of your choice

❶ Mix ingredients in proportion desired
❷ Apply to surface

---

To sum it up, keep sweeping to a minimum when cleaning floors; opt for the mop instead. Take precautions when changing your vacuum cleaner bag. Use natural oils and beeswax when necessary, and stick with the basic formulas when removing stains. Following these procedures will not only prove perfectly satisfactory for the job, but will keep your home environmentally safe.

# Chapter 6

# MASTERING YOUR MISERY OVER METALS

Metal is a hard substance, and most people assume it is just as hard to properly clean—at least without the aid of strong toxic commercial polishes. Not so. The potent acids that these products contain can be matched by implementing naturally acidic substances such as lemons or vinegar. Add a measure of abrasion, such as what can be achieved with salt, and you have a competent cleaner.

---

⊠ **Caution:** Give the selected formula time to do its work. If you try to help it along by using a scouring pad, you will scratch the surface. Stick to a rag or sponge.

---

## Ideas for Aluminum

There are a number of worthwhile items to use when cleaning aluminum. Citrus is usually adequate in itself. Try 2 or 3 lemon or lime halves, or 1 grapefruit cut in quarters. Place them and the tarnished item in a pan full of water and boil on low heat until the discoloration disappears. Or, if needed, use this process to detarnish the pan itself.

## Suggested Aluminum Cleaner 1

- 2 or 3 lemon or lime halves, or 1/4 grapefruit
- Water

❶ Place fruit and tarnished item in pan full of water
❷ Boil on low heat until the discoloration disappears

This same method can be employed by using several freshly cut stalks of rhubarb, apple peelings, or sliced tomatoes. Just make certain the areas to be cleaned are completely submerged in the water.

## Suggested Aluminum Cleaner 2

- Several freshly cut stalks of rhubarb or apple peelings or sliced tomatoes
- Water

● Follow above instructions

⊠ **Caution:** It is not recommended that you use washing soda, baking soda, or borax on aluminum on a continued basis. These substances will subject this metal to discoloration and eventual deterioration.

⊠ **Caution:** Higher than normal concentrations of aluminum in brain tissue have been associated with Alzheimer's disease. Although it has not been proven to be the cause, it might not be wise to rely heavily on using aluminum cookware. When it is heated, a certain amount of vapor from the aluminum will be released into the air. For this reason, it would probably be safer to use the formulas below for cleaning this metal:

Form a paste out of cornstarch and alum in a 50-50 ratio. Rub it on with a moist sponge and allow to dry. Rinse in hot water, then rub with a clean cloth until shiny.

## Suggested Aluminum Cleaner 3

• Cornstrach
• Alum

❶ Make a paste with equal amounts of both ingredients
❷ Rub on with moist sponge
❸ Allow to dry
❹ Rinse in hot water
❺ Then rub with clean cloth until shiny

Another effective method involves a cream of tartar and vinegar mixture. Be conservative enough with the vinegar to maintain a firm paste. Use a cloth or sponge to rub in the formula. Wash it off with hot water only after it has thoroughly dried. Then dry with a clean rag.

## Suggested Aluminum Cleaner 4

• Cream of tartar
• Vinegar

❶ Mix ingredients using just enough vinegar to make firm paste
❷ Rub into surface with cloth or sponge
❸ Allow to thoroughly dry
❹ Wash off with hot water
❺ Dry with clean rag

---

❋ **Handy hint:** When you rub aluminum, apply horizontal or vertical motion instead of a circular one. This will help maintain a uniform appearance. (In reality, this is a good practice when cleaning other surfaces because most everything, even if not obvious, has a grain or texture that runs in a specific direction.)

## The Solution for Shiny Chrome

Usually you only need to rub chrome with a soft, damp cloth and polish it with a dry one. All you will ever possibly require in the way of a cleaner is baking soda, a lemon rind or vinegar. If you use baking soda, make it into a paste with water and rub it in with a cloth. Then rinse thoroughly using warm water and finish off by polishing. Or use the inner portion of a lemon half (the portion that is white). Rub it in and rinse. Or douse a sponge with vinegar, apply, and rinse.

---

## Suggested Chrome Cleaner 1

• Baking soda
• Water

❶ Make a paste by combining the ingredients
❷ Rub in with cloth
❸ Rinse thoroughly with warm water
❹ Polish dry with a dry cloth

---

## Suggested Chrome Cleaner 2

• Lemon half

❶ Rub inner part of fruit on surface
❷ Rinse

---

## Suggested Chrome Cleaner 3

• Vinegar

❶ Apply with sponge
❷ Rinse

---

## Getting Brazen with Bronze, Brass and Copper

Each of these metals can receive the same basic treatment since they are all similar in nature. Both brass and bronze are composed partially of copper.

The dependable juice of the lemon and table salt come into play here, too. Make a paste from equal parts of each (1 to 2 tablespoons is a good rule of thumb). Use a sponge to apply. Rinse with hot water and follow up by polishing dry with a soft rag. Flour can also be added to the formula and vinegar can be substituted for lemon juice. Baking soda or cream of tartar in paste form will also work. Or for a quicker solution, just rub a freshly cut lemon half into some salt and apply. This is especially convenient for small ornate pieces that are difficult to maneuver around. For best results, allow the formula to remain on the surface for 5 minutes, then rinse with warm water and dry.

---

**Suggested Bronze, Brass, and Copper Cleaner 1**

• 1 or 2 tablespoons lemon juice or vinegar
• 1 or 2 tablespoons salt
• 1 teaspoon flour (optional)

❶ Make a paste by combining ingredients
❷ Apply with sponge
❸ Rinse with hot water
❹ Polish dry with soft rag

---

**Suggested Bronze, Brass, and Copper Cleaner 2**

• 1 or 2 tablespoons baking soda
• 1 or 2 tablespoons cream of tartar

● Follow above instructions

---

**Suggested Bronze, Brass, and Copper Cleaner 3**

• Lemon half
• Salt

❶ Rub fruit into salt
❷ Rub on surface
❸ For best results, allow formula to remain for 5 minutes
❹ Then rinse with warm water
❺ Polish dry

---

If you have ever been stricken with insomnia, you probably know that hot milk serves as a good sedative. But did you know that it's also an efficient copper-based metal cleaner? All you have to do is place the stained article in a pan of 1 part water and 1 part milk, and simmer for approximately 1 hour. Buttermilk or tomato juice can also be used.

---

**Suggested Bronze, Brass, and Copper Cleaner 4**

• 1 part milk, buttermilk or tomato juice
• 1 part water

❶ Pour ingredients into pan
❷ Place metal article in pan
❸ Simmer for 1 hour

---

And those who are becoming bored with the same ingredients need only to reach into their pantry for a bottle of catsup, tabasco sauce or worcestershire sauce. These work, too. Rub into the metal aggressively with a sponge, rinse with hot water and dry.

---

## Suggested Bronze, Brass, and Copper Cleaner 5

• Catsup, tabasco sauce, or worcestershire sauce

❶ Rub into metal aggressively with sponge
❷ Rinse in hot water
❸ Polish dry

---

❋ **Handy hint:** For heavily tarnished items, allow any formula to remain in contact with the metal for a few hours or overnight.

---

The one drawback to cleaning these metals with acidic ingredients is that retarnishing can rapidly take place. To avoid this, wash in water and a vegetable-oil-based soap after the cleaner has done its job.

Lacquered brass or bronze will not require anything more than dusting and an occasional washing with a vegetable-oil-based soap. Make sure the water is lukewarm. Hot water (and other cleaning ingredients) will damage the lacquer. When done, rinse and dry.

---

**Suggested Bronze, Brass, and Copper Cleaner 6**

• Vegetable-oil-based liquid soap
• Lukewarm water

❶ For lacquered metals, wash with ingredients
❷ Rinse
❸ Dry

---

## All the Gold that Glitters

For gold articles, reach into the medicine cabinet and get your tube of toothpaste. (Make sure it's white and not one of the multi-colored kinds.) Just rub some on the metal with your fingers, then rinse thoroughly in hot water and polish to a dry shine.

---

**Suggested Gold Cleaner 1**

• White toothpaste

❶ Rub on surface with fingers
❷ Rinse thoroughly in hot water
❸ Polish dry

---

❋ **Handy hint:** If you don't cherish the thought of using bare fingers for this job, apply with a sponge. But believe it or not, the body oils from your skin combine with the toothpaste to make a more effective cleaner.

If gold jewelry is your concern, you can soak these valuables in a glass jar containing a mixture of baking soda, toothpaste and warm water. Just use enough water to cover the tarnished items, add a few blobs of toothpaste, and a small handful of soda. Then screw on the lid and shake vigorously. Rinse thoroughly and polish dry. For particularly challenging jobs, let the jewelry remain in the jar for several hours first.

---

## Suggested Gold Cleaner 2

- Handful baking soda
- Several squirts of toothpaste
- Warm water

❶ Mix ingredients in glass jar
❷ Place small items such as jewelry in jar
❸ Screw on lid and shake vigorously
❹ Rinse thoroughly
❺ Polish dry

---

## More than a Silver Lining

Before worrying about returning the luster to silver, think about how it can be kept from losing its shine in the first place. When it's not being used, it should be wrapped snugly in a soft cloth or felt and stored in a dark place. Air and light will promote tarnish.

So much for the prevention; now for the cure. One of the rather fascinating solutions for achieving clean silver centers around aluminum foil and the process known as electrolysis. Place the silver into a big pan of water with a sheet of aluminum foil on the bottom and add 2 or 3 tablespoons of cream of tartar. If cream of tartar is not available, you can substitute baking soda and table salt. Heat under a flame and the work will do itself. As if by magic, within a short time (probably only several minutes), the aluminum foil will gradually attract all of the impurities! Then rinse the silver object(s) and polish dry to bring to a shine. You can also substitute washing soda for the baking soda/salt combination. For larger items, fill your sink with hot water, then add the foil and a few handfuls of salt.

You may wonder why you can't just forgo the foil and use an aluminum pan instead. You can, but then you will be left with a freshly tarnished pan.

---

**Suggested Silver Cleaner 1**

• Piece of aluminum foil
• 2 to 3 teaspoons of cream of tartar, or washing soda, or baking soda and salt

❶ Place foil at bottom of big pan of water
❷ Add ingredient(s) of choice
❸ Drop silver article(s) into big pan
❹ Heat under flame for a few minutes
❺ Then remove and rinse article(s)
❻ Polish dry

---

⊠ **Caution:** The above procedure is not advised for antique silver finishes, hollowware or items that might be bound with glue such as flat silver with hollow handles.

> ⊠ **Caution:** It is not advisable to soak silver pieces that are glued together.

White toothpaste also works well for silver. Apply it the same way suggested for cleaning gold. In addition, silver can be soaked in lemon or lime juice, or vinegar and milk. Lacquered silver requires only luke warm water and a vegetable-oil-based liquid soap.

---

**Suggested Silver Cleaner 2**

• White toothpaste

● Apply as you would when cleaning gold

---

**Suggested Silver Cleaner 3**

• Lemon or line juice or vinegar and milk

● Soak in one of the above ingredients

---

## Putting Up With Pewter

There are several interesting ingredients that can be used to clean this alloy. One answer is to grind up some sticks of blackboard chalk and mix with alcohol to form a paste. Apply the paste as you would for other metals. Vodka or brandy can be substituted for the alcohol. You can also mix up a flour/salt/vinegar paste.

## Suggested Pewter Cleaner 1

• Chalk
• Alcohol

❶ Grind chalk sticks
❷ Mix with alcohol to form paste
❸ Apply as you would for other metals

## Suggested Pewter Cleaner 2

• Flour
• Salt
• Vinegar

❶ Mix ingredients to form paste
❷ Apply as you would for other metals

In addition, a paste made of olive oil, vinegar and fine rottenstone is effective. Just add a handful of rottenstone and a few drops of vinegar to the oil until you have a reasonably thick consistency. Rub it into the pewter with your fingers.

## Suggested Pewter Cleaner 3

• Olive oil
• Vinegar
• Rottenstone (fine)

❶ Add a handful of rottenstone and a few drops of vinegar to the oil until you have a reasonably thick paste
❷ Rub into surface with fingers

Another idea is to rescue a wedge of cabbage, perhaps from the salad you are planning for dinner, moisten and salt the freshly cut end, and rub it onto the pewter.

---

**Suggested Pewter Cleaner 4**

• Cabbage
• Salt

❶ Moisten freshly cut end of cabbage
❷ Then add salt
❸ Rub onto surface

---

In any case, allow whatever formula you've chosen to remain on the surface until it has dried. Then use a clean cloth to polish, wash with a vegetable-oil-based liquid soap, rinse, and dry.

---

⊠ **Caution:** It is not recommended that you use washing soda, baking soda or borax on pewter. Due to its soft nature, this metal is vulnerable to scratch damage from the heavier abrasives.

---

## No Need to be an "Iron Man"

The trouble with iron is that it rusts. This process of oxidation can be avoided by not allowing an iron surface to remain moist.

As with aluminum, rhubarb is a good iron cleaner. (See the section on aluminum above.) Or throw some hay into a rusty skillet or pot and add water along with approximately 1/4 cup of vinegar. Set the utensil on a flame and boil until the rust has disappeared. Repeat if necessary.

## Suggested Iron Cleaner 1

• Several freshly cut stalks of rhubarb

❶ Place rhubarb and tarnished item in pan full of water
❷ Boil on low heat until the discoloration disappears

## Suggested Iron Cleaner 2

• Hay
• Water
• 1/4 cup of vinegar

❶ Throw hay into rusty skillet or pot
❷ Add water and vinegar
❸ Set on a flame and boil until rust disappears
❹ Repeat if necessary

If you like, take a cloth that has been dipped in vegetable oil and rub it vigorously on rusty areas. For an iron rust-protectant, coat the clean surface with vegetable oil.

## Suggested Iron Cleaner 3

• Vegetable oil

❶ Dip cloth in vegetable-oil
❷ Rub vigorously on rusty areas

Fine emery cloth can also be applied to iron. Gently rub the surface, then wipe with a soft cloth that has been dipped in olive oil.

## Suggested Iron Cleaner 4

• Fine emery cloth
• Olive oil

❶ Gently rub surface with emery cloth
❷ Dip soft cloth or rag in olive oil
❸ Then wipe surface

# The Secret About Stain(less) Steel

It's an interesting thing about stainless steel—it doesn't remain stainless and must be cleaned just as any other substance. In fact, some of the less expensive varieties actually streak and stain quite easily.

But stainless steel sinks, toasters and other items can just as easily be cleaned with a few of the faithful standbys. Rub on a lemon juice and salt solution, or a paste made from baking soda or borax and water. Or use alcohol. Vinegar also works. In addition, you can use white toothpaste as you would to clean other metals. Usually, however, all that is required is the utilization of a damp sponge followed by a dry cloth.

## Suggested Stainless Steel Cleaner 1

• Lemon juice
• Salt

❶ Mix ingredients
❷ Rub on surface with cloth

---

**Suggested Stainless Steel Cleaner 2**

• Baking soda or borax
• Water

● Follow above instructions

---

**Suggested Stainless Steel Cleaner 3**

• Alcohol, vinegar, or white toothpaste

● Rub onto surface with cloth

---

## Knowing What to Do About Nickel

Nickel, a hard silver-white metal that darkens if not cleaned often, is commonly used as plating for copper or steel. A vegetable-oil-based soap and water should be all that is necessary to keep it shiny. If you require more, mix a small amount of chalk dust or other fine abrasive with alcohol. In either case, rinse afterwards and polish dry.

---

**Suggested Nickel Cleaner 1**

• Vegetable-oil-based liquid soap
• Water

❶ Mix ingredients
❷ Clean as you would other items
❸ Rinse
❹ Polish dry

## Suggested Nickel Cleaner 2

• Chalk
• Alcohol

❶ Grind stick of chalk
❷ Then follow above instructions

## The Truth About Tin

Bread pans, piepans and other such kitchen accessories that are composed of tin need only be washed in vegetable-oil-based soap and water. But they must be rinsed and dried thoroughly to prevent rust. If you scrub with heavy abrasives, you may remove the tin, which is in reality only a coating. Although you'll want to make sure they are clean, there is really no point in keeping these articles shiny. Darker surfaces absorb the heat better and are therefore more efficient for cooking.

## Suggested Tin Cleaner 1

• Vegetable-oil-based liquid soap
• Water

❶ Mix ingredients
❷ Wash surface
❸ Rinse thoroughly
❹ Dry thoroughly

To eliminate grease spots, wash tinware in a solution of 1/4 cup of washing soda and 1 quart of water. If you're faced with rust, rub a raw potato in a mild abrasive such as cream of tartar and then apply it to the surface. For burned-on food residue, fill with water, add a small amount of baking soda, and boil for no more than 5 minutes.

---

## Suggested Tin Cleaner 2

- 1/4 cup washing soda
- 1 quart water

● Follow above instructions

---

## Suggested Tin Cleaner 3

- 1 raw potato
- Cream of tartar

❶ Rub potato in cream of tartar
❷ Then apply to surface
❸ Rinse thoroughly
❹ Dry thoroughly

---

## Suggested Tin Cleaner 4

- Baking soda
- Water

❶ Fill tin cookware with water
❷ Add small amount of soda
❸ Boil for 5 minutes
❹ Wash as usual

---

In general, the dependable common metal cleaners include lemon, vinegar, toothpaste and chalk. These materials can be just as effective as any metal cleaner on the market. There is one other ingredient that can be used for metal cleaning: wood ashes. If you own an active fireplace, you'll have no trouble gathering a handful. Just rub them onto the tarnished metal with the aid of a moistened sponge until it comes clean.

# Chapter 7

# NOTHING TO GET BROKEN UP OVER

How about this formula? A truckload of silica combined with a few wheelbarrows of lime and soda ash, and melted at a high temperature. This is not a suggestion for a home cleaner. Actually, this combination creates a very common product: glass.

## Getting a Clear Idea About Glass

Even with problem streaks, glass has a number of advantages. Although it is breakable, it does not peel, fade, rot, burn, blister or rust. It matches any decor, never goes out of style, and doesn't even need to be painted. Besides, glass can be cleaned quickly and easily if one uses the right method.

"Sure," you say, "I've heard that one before." But there are a couple of facts about cleaning glass windows you might not be aware of. Fact no. 1: Don't use formulas with a high soap content. Soapy residue easily builds up and remains on the surface, only to be smeared every time you face another cleaning job. Furthermore, a soapy film attracts dust, lint and other matter, which itself can create streaks unless it is adequately removed by using an efficient cleaning formula. Streaks can be produced by washing windows when the sun is shining on them because the cleaning formula will dry too fast.

As for the second fact, use the proper tool to finish the job: a squeegee. And while you're at it, go for the best. Purchase one from a janitorial supply store. For the typical home, 10 inches to 12 inches is a comfortable width. This size blade will accommodate most panes. If your windows are composed of large sections of glass, you may be better off with an 18 inch blade. But remember, there are always areas where only a smaller tool is going to fit. For high areas, make sure you have an extension handle to add to your squeegee.

---

❋ **Handy hint:** Make sure the rubber blade of your squeegee extends slightly beyond its frame on both ends. That way you will avoid scraping the metal of your tool into window and door frames.

---

Now for some simple formulas to go along with this tool. How about the simplest of all—2 parts hydrogen and 1 part oxygen? That's right, $H_2O$. If the job is light, plain cool water by itself will be perfectly ample. Just add to a spray bottle, shake, and spray. Then distribute thoroughly along the glass with a sponge and put your squeegee to work.

If you require a stronger cleaner, one idea is to add 1/2 cup of vinegar or lemon juice to 2 cups of water. Another solution is to use a cup of cooled black tea and 3 or 4 tablespoons of vinegar or lemon juice. If you are dealing with an excessive amount of grime, add 1/4 teaspoon of vegetable-oil-based liquid soap to one of these formulas. There is no reason to use the soap, however, unless absolutely necessary.

## Suggested Glass Cleaner 1

- 1/2 cup vinegar or lemon juice
- 2 cups water
- 1/4 teaspoon vegetable-oil-based liquid soap (optional)

❶ Combine ingredients in bucket or spray bottle
❷ Wipe with sponge
❸ Dry with squeegee

## Suggested Glass Cleaner 2

- 1 cup cooled black tea
- 3 to 4 tablespoons vinegar or lemon juice
- 1/4 teaspoon vegetable-oil-based liquid soap (optional)

● Follow above instructions

Many prefer alcohol for cleaning windows. And there is no doubt that it is an excellent glass cleaner. Use about 1/4 cup for every quart of water. Alcohol is especially desirable if you happen to be washing windows in freezing temperatures. It can also help remove a waxy residue that can accumulate on the surface from the extended use of certain chemical glass cleaners.

## Suggested Glass Cleaner 3

- 1/4 cup alcohol
- 1 quart water

● Follow above instructions

Resist the temptation to wipe away those little spots of moisture. Let them evaporate. There will be nothing left but sparkling glass minus the streaks.

If you require or prefer a measure of abrasiveness because of thick grime or mineral build-up, pour a few tablespoons of table salt, cornstarch, or borax and 1/2 cup of cold water in a wide-mouthed container. Dab a sponge or a soft cotton rag into the solution and apply to the window. Then follow up with one of the above formulas and finish with your squeegee.

---

**Suggested Glass Cleaner 4**

• Several tablespoons salt, cornstarch, or borax
• 1/2 cup cold water

❶ Combine ingredients in bucket
❷ Apply with sponge or rag
❸ Then use one of the other formulas above

---

A few annoying lines produced by the squeegee will probably still remain. Don't use a cloth to wipe them. That will only leave a wider mark and may even deposit lint. Instead, use a finger. That's right! Your fingers, ordinarily oily by nature, should be free of oil because your hands will have caught a lot of drip from the solution. So before your body oil has a chance to rise back through your pores, use one of your freshly dried fingers to gently stroke away at the unsightly marks.

If you are called on to remove labels, decals or paint spots from a window, vigorously rub with a solution of hot vinegar and washing soda, or apply linseed oil. These ingredients will soften them, therefore making them easier to separate from the surface. You may have to use a razor blade to complete the job, but proceed with caution if doing so.

## Suggested Glass Cleaner 5

- Hot vinegar
- Washing soda

❶ Combine ingredients
❷ Vigorously rub paints spots, labels or decals stuck on surface
❸ Allow to sit until softened
❹ Scrape off

## Suggested Glass Cleaner 6

- Linseed oil

❶ Vigorously rub paints spots, labels or decals stuck on surface
❷ Allow to sit until softened
❸ Scrape off

⊠ **Caution:** Don't use a dry cloth to scrub dirty glass. You might scratch the surface. For this same reason, the glass must be kept wet if you're using a razor blade to remove foreign substances from a window.

✱ **Handy hint:** When using your squeegee, avoid contact with walls and other rough surfaces. You want to keep the rubber blade as sharp as possible.

## Other Glass Items

That takes care of the windows. But you'd be surprised at the number of other glass items in a home. Mirrors, skylights, shelving, tabletops, light fixtures, and partitions are often just as common as windows. For these items, you won't need a squeegee. It will either be impractical for the job (as in the case of light fixtures, which are small and curved), or streaking won't be a major factor (as in the case of shelving, which will be largely hidden by the items occupying them). All you will need to do is apply one of the formulas suggested above with a sponge or rag.

---

❀ **Handy hint:** Skylights are very low-maintenance. The outside may never require washing and the inside needs it only occasionally at most.

---

Something else you may not have considered is stained glass. But unless it is extremely ornate in design, it won't pose as big of a problem as most glass surfaces. A little dusting is all that's usually required because it doesn't show the dirt as bad.

## Mirror, Mirror, Moisture and All

Actually, you might be wondering why a squeegee is not recommended for cleaning mirrors. There's no doubt that it would be just as effective as on glass panels, but a high amount of moisture should not be applied to mirrors. Some of this moisture can work its way into the mirror and turn its edges black. Just use a cloth or sponge dampened in the solution of your choice and wipe. In all likelihood, however, plain warm water and a soft cloth will be all that is necessary.

❀ **Handy hint:** Put a dab of glycerin on a wet rag or sponge and wipe onto your bathroom mirror before you shower. This will prevent the mirror from fogging.

And there you have it. No one has to shatter your dreams about having clean glass. Just use basic, easy-to-acquire ingredients, avoid soap whenever possible, and don't forget to finish the job with a squeegee.

# Chapter 8

# NO NEED TO CLIMB THE WALLS

Walls are often taken for granted—and they get quite a bit more wear than you probably ever realized. They're leaned against, pushed on, run into, and marked on, not to mention being adorned with sentimental possessions of all kinds. With all of this abuse, they fully deserve their share of cleaning attention.

The method you use for this purpose will vary according to the material(s) of which the wall is made. Most any of the general home-brew solutions mentioned earlier (contained in a plastic bucket), along with an additional empty bucket, a sponge and a cleaning cloth will take care of hard-surfaced walls whether it's textured, paneled, blocked, vinyl or whatever. Just apply the cleaner with the sponge and wipe dry with your cloth. Use the empty bucket to wring your sponge when it fills with dirt.

---

⊠ **Caution:** Don't use excessive abrasiveness on enamel surfaces unless absolutely necessary. It may dull the gloss.

---

## A Word About Wallpaper

For wallpaper that's badly soiled, consult Chapter 3. But lightly going over unsightly areas with a stick of chalk and then brushing clean will often take care of smudges on wallpaper. You might also consider a brown art store eraser. Another idea, believe it or not, is to rub with a slice of stale bread.

If the stain is greasy, place a piece of blotting paper over the area and press with a warm iron. Repeat as many times as necessary.

---

## Suggested Wallpaper Cleaner 1

• 1 stick of chalk

❶ Mark over stained areas
❷ Then brush clean

---

## Suggested Wallpaper Cleaner 2

• Brown art store eraser

● Follow above instructions

---

## Suggested Wallpaper Cleaner 3

• 1 slice stale bread

● Follow above instructions

---

## Lightening the Wall-Cleaning Burden

Here are some suggestions for making wall cleaning easier:

■ Before applying even a drop of cleaning solution to your dirty surfaces, give them the dry sponge. You'd be surprised the amount of loose dust and debris that can be picked up using one of these handy gadgets. They are great on most any surface, from wallpaper to painted walls to ceilings.

■ Go over all the baseboards with a vacuum cleaner or at least a damp rag, before you begin with the walls. You will pick up a lot of hair, dirt, spiders, and other such debris that can easily build up on a rag and certainly be difficult to dig out of a sponge. You don't want to face such an annoyance when you are right in the middle of washing down the second or third wall.

■ Vacuuming textured wall coverings before you apply any cleaner will remove dust that may be resting in the design pattern.

■ You will be much better off using plastic buckets rather than ones made of metal. Metal is prone to sweat, and it can nick furniture and walls if you're not careful.

■ When cleaning wallpaper, follow the flow of the design.

■ Start your cleaning from the top and work your way down.

■ Work in sections that are comfortable for you. A 3 by 3 foot area is a good rule-of-thumb.

■ It's better to lighten up. Putting too much pressure on the sponge will create an excessive amount of dripping.

■ Keep your drying cloth dry when finishing up enameled walls. This kind of surface shows wipe marks.

■ Wash an entire surface before you worry about heavy stains. They just might come off the first time around.

## The Fifth Wall

You have often heard the expression "staring at the four walls." But if you're lying in bed, you might just find yourself staring at what could easily be called a fifth wall—the ceiling.

The bad news is that ceilings are awkward to clean. The good news: They don't take near the abuse of their vertical counterparts, and therefore don't have to be cleaned often—perhaps only once every few years.

When faced with this endeavor, it is probably better to just dry sponge such surfaces and knock down or vacuum any cobwebs you find in the corners. Ceiling paints are usually not very washable. Don't forget to remove the light fixture diffusers before you begin. In fact, what a better time to clean *them*, too.

In the event you are faced with water stains from a leaking roof, apply hydrogen peroxide. Hopefully, long before then you will have patched your roof.

Even wall cleaning doesn't have to be a threat to your patience or your environment. All that is necessary is to invest a reasonable amount of time, be fully aware of the kind of surface(s) you are dealing with, and stick to environmentally friendly formulas.

# Chapter 9

# MANAGING MISCELLANEOUS AND DIFFICULT JOBS

There are always those special cleaning chores that must be done once in a while, or sometimes when you least suspect it—and certainly never when you want it. Some, in fact, are easy to neglect.

## Watching Out for Window Ware

It is often quite easy to forget about drapes. But they require attention, too. On an occasion when you are vacuuming the carpet, you may as well go ahead and run over them with dust brush attachment of your vacuum cleaner. This doesn't mean you have to do them every time, though.

You can also freshen drapes that aren't dirty enough to be cleaned with the vacuum cleaner by tossing them in the clothes dryer and allowing them to tumble a short time on a cool setting. Just make sure all of the hooks are removed before proceeding.

---

☒ **Caution:** Don't put fiberglass drapes in the dryer. Some of the fibers will flake off and remain, only to work their way into your next load of laundry.

---

---

❀ **Handy hint:** To protect drapes when cleaning the floor beneath them, hook a coat hanger on the rod and slip the bottom portion through it.

---

Cleaning blinds does not have to be a tough job if you keep up with them. Go over them at least once every month. Close them before you begin and use a lambswool duster. When you're finished, close them in the other direction and hit them again. They can also be vacuumed with the appropriate attachment.

When blinds have to be washed, do it outside. It will be a much messier job in the bathtub, or worse, while they're still on the window. Lay them on an old blanket, drop cloth, or other such article to protect them from damage, preferably on a slanted surface, and use one of the general environmentally safe cleaning formulas. Scrub in the same direction as the slats on both sides. Then rinse.

---

❀ **Handy hint:** Before you rinse your blinds, have a place prepared to hang them (such as a clothes line) until they dry.

---

A dry sponge is probably all you will require for window shades. Cleaning them, especially if they have aged, probably won't do much for their looks, because they are prone to discoloration from the sun.

## Producing Cleaner Trash

You may not be able to manufacture cleaner garbage, but you can control the cleanliness of the surfaces it comes in contact with. Ap proximately once a month, at one of those brief moments when your trash containers are freshly empty, wash them inside and out. Use lemon juice (to help cut sticky messes and to serve as a scent) and borax (as an abrasive and disinfectant). The problem of dirty trash containers can be reduced considerably, however, by taking care to line them with plastic bags. This may be a bit more costly, but it's worth the saving in time and aggravation.

---

## Suggested Trash Container Cleaner

• Lemon juice
• Borax

❶ Mix ingredients in quantity desired
❷ Wash interior and exterior surface

---

❋ **Handy hint:** If your trash befouls the air before you have a chance to remove it, just sprinkle a little baking soda in the container.

---

## A Matter of Mat Cleaning

Since mats do their part in keeping dirt confined (if your family uses them), they deserve to be cleaned once in a while. In fact, they demand to be cleaned, because they'll quit functioning efficiently if they're not.

The easiest way to accomplish this is to keep them vacuumed. You should do this once a week, when you're doing the floors. If they've become excessively dirty, hose them down, scrub with a water and lemon juice cleaner, and rinse thoroughly.

To speed up drying, you can use a squeegee to remove the majority of water, then hang them up to dry.

---

⊠ **Caution:** Use an old squeegee for this purpose. You may dull or damage the blade on a new one, and it won't be properly effective for cleaning windows.

---

## Fulfilling Your Filter-Cleaning Duties

Mats are not the only items that work for you. Don't overlook filters. They need attention, too. Heating and air conditioner filters require frequent replacement or cleaning, or they'll stop functioning. You'll then have a higher dust count in the indoor air, your equipment will be working harder, and utility bills will increase faster than the cost of living.

If you have washable filters, take them outside and hose them down. Use a lemon juice and water solution if you feel you need a cleaner to supplement your work. Allow them to dry and return them to their compartment. They may also be vacuumed.

If you own a washer and dryer, don't forget about their filters. Clean them every time they are used to maintain optimum appliance efficiency. Washing machine filters should be washed at the sink; clothes dryer filters can be dealt with by pulling off the layer of lint by hand. You can also run your vacuum cleaner hose over a dryer filter if it's handy at the time. While you're at it, clean out the area around the filter.

## Exhausting Dust from Exhaust Fans

Exhaust fans are often overlooked. Hopefully you have one in both the bathroom and the kitchen.

Even they must be cleaned occasionally. The cover plate can be removed and placed in a sink full of hot water and a vegetable-oil-based soap. While it is soaking, you can wipe out the exhaust opening with a solution of borax and water. The motor unit can also be removed and brushed off. But don't expose it to water—this could be harmful to the mechanism.

---

## Suggested Exhaust Fan Cleaner 1

• Vegetable-oil-based soap
• Hot water

❶ Place ingredients in sink
❷ Remove exhaust fan cover plate
❸ Soak
❹ Wipe off and dry

---

## Suggested Exhaust Fan Cleaner 2

• Borax
• Water

❶ Mix ingredients
❷ Use to wipe out exhaust opening

---

## Don't Duck Out on Duct Cleaning

Even your air ducts require cleaning attention (if you own a central heating and/or air conditioning system). In fact, they can quickly become one of the most contaminated areas of the house, because virtually every bit of matter that's loose in the air within your walls eventually circulates through them.

Air ducts also represent just about the most inaccessible area to clean. About all you can do yourself is vacuum the grill plates. Or you can remove and clean them, and then while the opening is accessible, run your vacuum hose as far up into the ducts as possible. It's recommended that you call a professional for this job on an annual basis. A professional service will also see that the blower, furnace, and air coils are cleaned. Just as with clean filters, clean ducts not only mean less debris circulating through the house, but better heating and cooling efficiency, and therefore lower electric bills.

## Cleaning Other Heating and Air Conditioning Devices

For those with portable air conditioning and heating units, remember that they require attention, too. Wiping the outside clean is easy enough, but checking the inside is more important. Mildew can grow inside air conditioning window units, and enclosed gas heaters will trap quite a lot of dust during the summer months. The more of this matter that's present, the more is released when the devices are used. Take off the protective covers and clean any accessible buildup off the interior sides, fan blades, heating elements or whatever applies. Play it safe, too, and unplug air conditioners (and/or electric heaters) before beginning your task. If you reside in an area near industrial pollution, heavy traffic, or the like, you may have to have window air conditioning units professionally steam cleaned once a year.

---

❉ **Handy hint:** Cover portable heaters and air conditioners with a drop cloth or other suitable material during the season they're not in use. This applies to electric baseboard heating and wall radiators as well.

If you use a fireplace, you can clean soot buildup with washing soda and water. Apply with an abrasive nylon pad. Vinegar can also be included in the formula. Or you can make a paste from salt, zinc oxide (available at your pharmacy), and water. Both options require a thorough rinse when you have finished scrubbing. The best bet is to have the fireplace and the chimney cleaned at the end of every season.

Wall radiators should be vacuumed periodically to avoid the formation of stains on the surfaces above and behind them created by rising dust. You can also use a lambswool duster instead of a vacuum cleaner. If nothing better, a brush can be used, but remember that while this will remove the dust from the object intended, it will also be stirred into the air.

For those who desire maximum mileage from their steam heat (and who doesn't?), you can also clean the radiator valves. Before the next heating season, unscrew the valves, place them in an enameled container, and add 2 tablespoons of washing soda with 2 quarts of water. Boil for several minutes. Then remove them, shake out the water, rinse, and return them to the radiator.

---

**Suggested Fireplace Cleaner 1**

• Washing soda
• Water
• Vinegar (optional)

❶ Combine ingredients
❷ Apply with abrasive nylon pad
❸ Rinse thoroughly

---

## Suggested Fireplace Cleaner 2

- Salt
- Zinc oxide
- Water

● Follow above instructions

---

## Controlling Stains with an Iron Hand

Removing starch buildup and discoloration from the bottom of your iron is simple. Wait until the iron has cooled and rub with a cloth soaked in diluted vinegar. Or sprinkle some salt on your ironing board and run over it a few times while the iron is warm. It's also a good idea to fill the reservoir of your steam iron with undiluted vinegar now and then to prevent corrosion and calcium deposits. When the vinegar is in, iron a rag, then iron again using water and, finally, flush out the reservoir.

---

## Suggested Clothes Iron Cleaner 1

- Vinegar

❶ Soak cloth in diluted vinegar
❷ Rub on bottom of cooled iron

---

## Suggested Clothes Iron Cleaner 2

- Salt

❶ Sprinkle on ironing board
❷ Run over it a few times while the iron is warm

## Where There is Fire

It's a wise idea to vacuum smoke detectors occasionally. If the circuitry becomes clogged with excessive dust, the unit may be rendered inoperative.

## Making Music With Alcohol

When you need to clean the keys of your piano or organ, try some rubbing alcohol. A few tablespoons in 1/4 cup of water is plenty. You may not enjoy the kind of music you make when wiping them, but they'll be clean. And rinsing won't be necessary because the alcohol quickly evaporates, leaving nothing trapped between the keys.

## Livening Up Lacquered Articles

To restore the luster to dull lacquered articles, dip them in warm water and either sour milk or lemon juice. Rub with a soft cloth. Allow to dry in a warm place and polish. For tougher jobs, apply a paste made of olive oil and flour. Rub in well, wipe off, then polish with a soft cloth.

## Unlocking the Problem of Rust

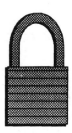

You can eliminate rust from padlocks by soaking them in vinegar. Vinegar can also be used instead of oil to loosen a lock that is stuck. In addition, other rusty objects can benefit from the application of vinegar.

## Shaking Off an Annoying Problem

Who has not had a salt shaker with a hopelessly stuck lid? Simply soak in hot vinegar for awhile. Not only will this loosen the tops, but the corrosive material that caused the problem will be easier to wash off. In more severe cases, add salt to the vinegar.

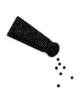

## Maintaining Your Resilience with Rubber Articles

Rubber articles such as boots, raincoats, hot water bottles, and ice packs can be kept clean by vegetable-oil-based soap and water. After cleaning, rinse with a cloth wrung from warm water, then either wipe them dry or allow them to dry in a cool, well-ventilated area.

## Getting Tough with Chemical Spills

It happens to the best of us. We try to be careful, but sometimes we find ourselves in a little more of a hurry than we should be, and spill a big batch of some richly colored household chemical (which was probably against our best interest to use in the first place). Suddenly there's an extra cleanup chore ahead of us. But it doesn't have to be as disastrous as Humpty Dumpty's great fall.

You should take action at once, especially if it's a big spill, and even more so if it's a potent substance. The first move is to reach for the kitty litter or cornstarch. Apply a generous

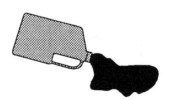

amount to the area and let it absorb what it can. When you've removed as much of the chemical as possible, cover what remains with a paste made from potter's clay and water. The clay must be left on the soiled area for at least 6 hours, perhaps more. Remove, then repeat the process several times if a stain lingers.

---

⊠ **Caution:** It's not recommended that the above cleaning formula be used if an industrial-strength chemical spill is involved. In such cases, you should consult the manufacturer of the product.

---

## Suggested Chemical Spill Cleaner

• Kitty litter or cornstarch
• Potter's clay
• Water

❶ Apply generous amount of kitty litter or corn starch to area
❷ Allow it to absorb as much of stain as possible
❸ Then remove it
❹ Cover what residue that remains with a potter's clay and water paste
❺ Allow to remain 6 hours or more
❻ Remove
❼ Repeat several times if necessary

---

That just about covers environmentally friendly cleaning in regard to the inside of your home. Now that you have a good grasp of what this kind of cleaning is all about, not only will you be successful in this aspect of cleaning, but you'll be placing much less strain on you and your family's immune systems—and you may even come up with some ideas of your own.

# Chapter 10

# NOTHING LIKE THE GREAT OUTDOORS

Actually, the interior of a home is not the only thing that needs attention. The outside must be maintained as well. Not only does this part of your home have a lot to do with the amount cleaning you must perform inside (more on this in the "Your Ounce of Prevention" section), but it is the portion that is seen first.

## Making a Clean Sweep

When you clean the exterior mats, it would also be a good time to perform some of those little extra outdoor chores, like sweeping the porch, the steps, and even the sidewalk. This is one time you won't have to be concerned about using a broom . Just make sure, of course, that the wind is with you so you won't allow any stirred-up debris to hit you in the face.

## Screens: Another Part of Window Washing

Glass is not the only surface to consider when washing windows. The screens eventually need attention too. In fact, it's often the screens that make windows appear dirty. They can become embedded with mud, dead bugs, bird droppings, tree sap and other plant debris. When it rains, some of these remains are washed are washed from the screens and wind up on the window panes.

When the need arises, remove the screens and lay them flat on a drop cloth or an old rug. Use a soft-bristled brush and a lemon juice or vinegar solution to clean them. When you are finished, hose them down, give them a few gentle taps to force loose the majority of water that will still be clinging to their surface, and allow them to dry in the sun. Meanwhile, there is no better time to wash the outside glass of all your windows.

If time is short, you can avoid taking them down by vacuuming them or lightly sweeping them with a broom or brush. Then wipe them down with a damp cloth. Needless to say, don't place excess pressure on them, or you'll be risking damage.

---

**Suggested Window Screen Cleaner**

- 1 part vinegar or lemon juice
- 1 part water

❶ Combine ingredients
❷ Apply with soft-bristled brush
❸ Rinse
❹ Give screens a few gentle taps
❺ Allow to dry in sun

---

## The Other Side of the Wall

There are not only two sides to every story, but two sides to every wall. Although they take a harsh beating from the elements, you might find an occasion to hose down aluminum siding, brick or wood that is unusually soiled. If any of these surfaces have been defaced, try using one of the formulas for stains. (See Chapter 3 for details.)

## Cleaning Up Motor Oil Spills

What driveway or garage floor has ever remained unsoiled? It is a fact of life that all automobiles, whether truck, van, or Rolls Royce, will spring a leak sooner or later, resulting in that annoying, ever-growing spot of oil. It makes you wish you had thought of keeping an oil pan underneath the engine crankcase—a good point to remember in the future. To handle this job, you'll need the following: A few teaspoons of washing soda, 1/4 teaspoon of vegetable-oil-based liquid soap, and either cornstarch, bran, oatmeal, stale bread crumbs, kitty litter, fuller's earth, sawdust, sand or concrete mix for an absorbent. Place enough of any of these absorbents to cover the spot, and allow it to absorb the grease. Then sweep it away. If the spill is fresh and large in volume, you'll have to make several applications. When you have eliminated all of the excess you can, mix the washing soda with 2 cups of hot water, add the soap, and pour it on the stain. Use a scrub brush for the final cleaning. Don't forget to take care in disposing of the used absorbent.

---

## Suggested Cleaners for Motor Oil Spills

- Several teaspoons washing soda
- 2 cups hot water
- 1/4 teaspoon vegetable-oil-based liquid soap
- Cornstarch, bran, oatmeal, stale bread crumbs, kitty litter, fuller's earth, sawdust, sand or concrete mix

❶ Completely cover the spot with cornstarch or other absorbent of your choice
❷ Allow it to absorb grease
❸ Then sweep away
❹ Repeat several times if necessary
❺ When excess oil has been absorbed, mix washing soda with hot water
❻ Add soap and pour on stain
❼ Clean with scrub brush

## Speaking of Automobiles

Maybe the family car is not technically a part of the house, but it has to be cleaned once in a while, too.

You can wash your car with that by-now-familiar vegetable-oil-based liquid soap. Just drop 1/8 to 1/4 cup in a container and add warm water. Mix until 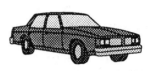 sudsy. Apply with a sponge, then rinse with the hose.

If you require additional help with chrome parts, use baking soda, a lemon rind or cider vinegar. (See Chapter 6 for details on cleaning chrome.)

If you live in a coastal region or cold climate where roads have to be salted in the winter, you'll inherit the additional problem of rust. Here's a trick that will help remove it from your car. Tear off several sheets of aluminum foil. Wet them with water and rub them only on the areas where the rust is.

---

⊠ **Caution:** Take care when working with aluminum foil. It will scratch chrome.

---

To prevent rust on your automobile, polish it with linseed oil and a rag. Also remember to keep any salt off the metal.

For removing tar, use 1 part lemon juice and 1 part linseed oil. Rub the solution onto the tar with a cloth. If you want to tone down scratches, rub with a crayon that matches the color the paint. Not only will this make the damage less conspicuous, the wax from the crayon will protect the exposed metal against rust.

You can use beeswax and linseed oil to wax your vehicle. (For details on preparing the wax, see Chapter 4.)

## Suggested Automobile Exterior Cleaner 1

- 1/8 to 1/4 cup vegetable-oil-based liquid soap
- Warm water

❶ Mix ingredients until sudsy
❷ Apply with sponge
❸ Then rinse

## Suggested Automobile Exterior Cleaner 2

- Baking soda
- Water

❶ Mix ingredients
❷ Use to clean chrome parts

## Suggested Automobile Exterior Cleaner 3

- 1 lemon rind, or cider vinegar

❶ Use either ingredient to clean chrome parts
❷ Rinse

## Suggested Automobile Exterior Cleaner 4

- Linseed oil

● To prevent rust, polish surface using rag

---

**Suggested Automobile Exterior Cleaner 5**

• Several sheets of aluminum foil

❶ Wet foil
❷ Rub them on areas of vehicle that are rusted

---

**Suggested Automobile Exterior Cleaner 6**

• 1 part lemon juice
• 1 part linseed oil

❶ Combine ingredients
❷ Use to remove tar by rubbing with cloth

---

**Suggested Automobile Exterior Cleaner 7**

• Crayon

● To make scratches less conspicuous, rub surface with crayon that matches the color of the paint

---

While we're at it, let's take a look at the inside. Most of us are aware of the odor released by vinyl upholstery. Scrubbing your seats will help, although it must be repeated at regular intervals. Use washing soda and boiling water or a vegetable-oil-based liquid soap and water. After about 2 years, however, this odor will begin to subside on its own.

## Suggested Automobile Interior Cleaner 1

- Washing soda
- Boiling water

❶ Combine ingredients
❷ Apply to vinyl upholstery with sponge or cloth

## Suggested Automobile Interior Cleaner 2

- Vegetable-oil-based liquid soap
- Water

● Follow above instructions

When one talks about the inside of a car, there is another area which qualifies: under the hood. Don't panic; you don't have to turn yourself into a mechanic. But there are a couple of simple maneuvers you can perform if you like.

The radiator can be cleaned with washing soda and boiling water. Use a brush to scrub on the mixture, then rinse off with a rag and hot water. If you really want to get serious, add a little baking soda and apply to the rest of the engine. Also, baking soda and a dab of water is an excellent combination to use for cleaning the battery terminals. Many "sluggish or dead batteries" are nothing more than the result of a loose connection due to acid buildup. Apply it with a brush, then watch it bubble and listen to it fizz as it does its work.

And there you have it. As you can see, environmentally friendly cleaning formulas and procedures are appropriate for use outside the home as well. They are safe and effective on most anything.

# Chapter 11

# ENERGY-SAVING TIPS

Tips on how to operate your home more efficiently and save money.

# Energy-Saving Tips

Not only do you want to maintain a clean home in an environmentally sound fashion, while saving as much money as you can, you also want to operate that home as inexpensively as possible. Here is a list of useful tips to help you in this endeavor.

## Water Heater

• Lower the thermostat on your water heater to no more than 120 º F. That setting provides comfortably hot water for most applications.

• Consider insulating the storage tank of your water heater, including the first six feet of the hot and cold water pipes connected to it. (But never cover the thermostat.) Heat traps can also be installed on the pipes, unless you have a model with built-in traps.

• It's a good idea to drain a quart of water from your hot-water storage tank every three months to remove sediment that can impede the transfer of heat. The procedure for doing this varies according to the model you own so check manufacturer's instructions.

• If you are purchasing a new water heater, make sure it is an energy-efficient model. If you are in an unshaded south-facing location, you may want to consider investing in a solar water heating system, which is more environmentally friendly.

## Heating and Cooling

• Keep air conditioning and heating filters clean or replace them as often as recommended.

• Check your ducts for air leaks. Avoid cloth-backed, rubber adhesive duct tape when sealing any holes you might find there as it tends to fail quickly. Hire a professional to make the repairs if necessary.

• If your ducts are not insulated, you can lose as much as 60% of your heated air before it reaches the register if they are routed through an attic or other unheated space.

• If using a fireplace, keep the flue damper closed tightly when not in use. As long as it is open, warm air is going to escape. In fact, it is equivalent to keeping a window wide open.

• Inspect the seal on the fireplace flue damper and make certain it is snug.

• The area around the fireplace hearth should be caulked.

• If your fireplace is never used, the chimney flue should be plugged and sealed.

• As a safety measure, it is a good idea to install carbon monoxide detectors in all homes with fuel-burning appliances. If the CO concentration reaches a dangerous level, an alarm will sound.

• Refrain from purchasing a bigger room air conditioner than is necessary for an area. It will not operate as efficiently as a smaller capacity unit because room window units function better if they run for relatively long periods of time rather than continually switching on and off. More lengthy run times will allow air conditioners to maintain a more constant temperature. (This principle also holds true for central air conditioning systems and need to be properly sized by a professional.)

• Portable fans used in conjunction with your window air conditioner will distribute the air more effectively while holding your power use down.

• Never place TV's or lamps near the air conditioning thermostat. They will generate heat the thermostat will sense, causing your air conditioner to run longer.

• Try to place room air conditioners on the north side of the house. That way they will be in the shade and will therefore consume as much as 10% less energy. (Planting shrubs or trees will help shade window units on other sides of the house, but make sure air flow to the unit is not blocked.)

• You may save as much as 50% on your cooling utility bill if you replace an older model air conditioner with a new one that is more energy-efficient.

• If you have a central air system, set the fan to turn off at the same time as the compressor. Use portable fans instead in individual rooms to provide continual circulation.

• Don't set your cooling thermostat lower than necessary when you turn on your air conditioner because it won't cool your house any faster.

• You may be able to save as much as 10% annually on heating and cooling bills by turning your thermostat back 10% to 15 % for eight-hour periods. If you would rather this be done automatically, consider installing an automatic setback or programmable thermostat. That way you can make adjustments for when you are asleep or are away at work.

## Insulating

• Add insulation to your attic. It is one of the most cost-effective ways to make your home more comfortable. Insulation should be of a rating between R-22 and R-49, depending upon the region where you live. Crawl spaces should also be insulated.

• As for new construction or home additions, R-11 to R-28 insulation (depending upon location) is recommended for exterior walls.

• In cathedral ceilings and on exterior walls, install higher-density insulation.

• One should check for air leaks around window frames, door frames, electrical switches and outlets, sill plates, chimney flashing, plumbing access, furnace flues, ducts, and attic entrances. All these areas should be properly sealed with weather stripping or caulking.

• Rubber gaskets can be installed behind switch plates and electrical outlets on exterior walls.

• If there are dirty spots in your insulation, this is a sign that air is penetrating there from holes. These holes can be sealed by stapling sheets of plastic over them and caulking the edges of the plastic.

• Attaching heavy-duty, clear plastic sheets to the inside of your windows during the winter months will cut down heat transference.

• Single-pane windows should be replaced with the double-pane variety or storm windows should be added. Storm windows (and doors) can deduce heat loss by from 25% to 50%.

## Appliances

• Rather than depend on your dishwasher's drying cycle, air dry dishes.

• Wash only full loads of clothes and dishes, but never overfill.

• Wash clothes with less water and cooler water. The load's energy use can be cut to as much as half by switching the machine's setting from hot to warm.

• Do not over-dry clothes.

• For the best appliance efficiency, the dryer's lint filter should be cleaned after every load.

• Your dryer vent should be inspected periodically for blockages, which will not only reduce the efficiency of the machine, but can become a fire hazard.

• Your might want to consider giving your dryer a rest and use an old-fashioned clothes line for drying your clothes. If weather does not permit, there are wind-up indoor clothes lines available.

• Don't keep your refrigerator or freezer colder than necessary. For the fresh food compartment a temperature of 37 $^{\circ}$ to 40 $^{\circ}$ F. is recommended and 5 $^{\circ}$ F. for the freezer section. Check the temperature by placing an appliance thermometer in a glass of water and keeping it in the center of the fridge for 24 hours. For the freezer, place a thermometer between frozen packages and take a reading after 24 hours.

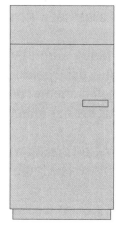

• Don't allow frost to build up to more than a quarter of an inch in manual-defrost refrigerators. Energy efficiency is decreased by this accumulation. Keep them defrosted regularly.

• Make certain the door seals on your refrigerator are adequately tight. You can test them by closing the door on a piece of paper that is half in and half out. If the paper can be pulled out easily, you might need to adjust the latch or the seal may need to be replaced.

• Cover foods and liquid in your refrigerator. Uncovered foods release moisture thereby forcing the compressor to work harder.

• If you are in the market for a new refrigerator, bear in mind that the top freezer models are more energy efficient than the side-by-side models. Also, models with ice-makers, as convenient as they are, are less efficient.

• If you plan to purchase a natural gas stove or range, look for a model with an automatic electric ignition system. That way you avoid a continually lit pilot that will consume more fuel.

• Make sure that flames of gas appliances burn blue. If they burn yellow or orange, burning is more inefficient and an adjustment is necessary. Consult the manufacturer, if not your local utility.

• When boiling water, use a covered pan or kettle. This will be faster and consume less energy.

• For small meals, consider using toaster ovens. A toaster oven uses a third to a half as much energy as a full-size oven.

• Energy can also be saved by the use of pressure cookers and microwaves, which considerably reduce cooking time.

## Lighting

• Replace incandescent light bulbs with fluorescent light bulbs. Ninety percent of an incandescent bulb's energy is thrown off as heat. Fluorescent lighting produces more light and lasts about 10 times longer. You might want to consider the latest thing: compact fluorescent light bulbs (CFLs), which—although considerably more expensive—are four times more efficient, while providing the same light level—and they have a long life (as much as 6 times longer). Halogen lamps should also be replaced. They produce excessive heat and are a potential fire hazard. For outdoor lighting, consider high-intensity discharge (HID) or low-pressure sodium lights.

• Turn lights off when not needed.

• Consider light dimmers and/or three-way lamps so the brightness of light can be readily controlled.

• Use task lighting rather than brightly lighting an entire room and focus the light where you require it.

• Try employing four-watt electro-luminescent and/ or minifluorescent night lights. They are more efficient than the incandescent variety.

• Use white- or light-colored, loose-weave curtains on windows to allow daylight to enter the room while your privacy is maintained. In warm-weather climates, keep in mind that white drapes, shades or blinds will reflect heat away from the house.

• Shades and curtains should be closed at night and opened during the day in the winter months.

• Use outdoor lights with motion sensors or photocell units so they will turn on only at night or when there is motion. A combination of both will save even more energy.

## Home/Office Equipment

• Don't forget about any office equipment you may be using in the home, such as computers, printers, scanners, and the like. Purchase energy efficient models and don't keep them on when not in use. Don't fail to take advantage of the power management feature of your computer.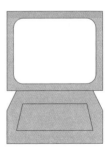

That way you can allow the stand by, sleep or hibernation mode to take effect whenever the equipment is idle for long enough. It will, of course, also shut off the monitor at appropriate times. If nothing more, manually turn off the monitor whenever you are not using it.

• To increase savings with a laptop, place the AC adapter on a power strip that can be turned off whenever appropriate. (The transformer in the AC adapter continuously draws power even when the laptop is not plugged into it.) Keep in mind that a laptop uses less energy than a desktop.

## Miscellaneous

• Keep your thermostat as low in winter and as high in summer as is comfortable.

• Don't use heated water from the tap when not necessary.

• Installing aerating, low-flow faucets and showerheads will reduce water consumption.

• Exhaust fans should be turned off within 20 minutes after you have finished bathing or cooking.

• TV's and many home electronics (and kitchen appliances) draw a certain amount of current even when not in operation. Unplug them when not in use for long periods of time, or better yet, plug them into power strips and turn them off whenever the equipment is not in use. A staggering 75% of the current used to power them is consumed while the devices are turned off!

## Clean, Green, Save—and More

You should now be fully apprised on how to keep your home clean and green, while saving lots of the long green as well. But there's more. You will discover many ways to make your cleaning job easier and save even more money in the section that follows.

# Chapter 12

# YOUR OUNCE OF PREVENTION

Make your environmentally friendly house-cleaning chores easier, while saving you even more money

# Your Ounce of Prevention

You don't need to be convinced that regular cleaning duties are enough of a challenge even when using the most basic ingredients. So before resuming your house-grooming campaign, even before picking up your next dust rag, it will be helpful to review the ways in which you can temper the hardship, while saving even more money.

## The Lowly Door Mat

The initial measure actually begins outside the house. According to the National Carpet Institute, an estimated 80% of dust and dirt in houses sneak in on the soles of the shoes. Believe it or not, one study disclosed that an average six-room dwelling in the city can accumulate as much as 40 pounds of dust a year!

So the first resort toward making your house-cleaning chores easier lies in the common door mat. While there is an initial cost, you will likely save more on cleaning supplies in the long run.

One should be placed at every entrance, including doorways leading in from the garage, where concrete dust, oil and grease, as well as dirt can pose a problem. Any mat will help, but the rougher in texture they are—and the bigger they are—the better.

Mats should be placed on the inside of the entrances too. A rugged nylon fiber type with rubber or vinyl backing is the best choice. The nylon actually produces a static charge, which pulls some of the particulate matter from shoes (and to a certain degree from clothes as well). They are also good absorbers of water and mud. Again, make certain they are large in size. And don't forget to encourage their use.

## Off With the Shoes

If you are meticulous enough, you may want to consider removing shoes when entering the house. They can be replaced with a pair reserved exclusively for indoors. You will not only avoid tracking in dirt, but save wear and tear on your better shoes and preserve more of your hard-earned funds.

## Clearing Out the Clutter

The next thing to do is to start simplifying the terrain. The rule here is "less is best." Although they are easy to accumulate, many items consuming space in the house are not needed or are no longer used. Discard some of those little kickknacks: the figurines and odd-shaped ornaments occupying shelves and tables. Don't let sentiment stand in the way. Once these "dust-catchers" are gone, you'll likely never miss them. You don't have to go as far as selling your prized vase, removing every extra stick of furniture or chucking out all the kid's toys. Just be reasonable. This is a chore that might become just as time-consuming as routine cleaning, but once it's done, it's done (at least for a long while). You'll eventually appreciate it because there will be fewer objects to dust and less territory to dust around.

Don't stop at what is in open view. Examine cabinets and drawers. You'll likely discover some old items that are no longer important to any of the family, or no longer serviceable—such as spray cans that fail to dispense their product, containers of dried up paint, and the like. This might also save you from a worse clean up chore, should a container get the opportunity to spring a leak and soil a cabinet shelf or drawer bottom. Even stored batteries can leak after a while and cause quite a mess.

---

✳ **Handy Hint:** Rather than sitting framed pictures on end tables or other furniture, combine them in one large frame and hang it on the wall.

---

Don't forget about one of the most popular hiding places of all—the closets. They can harbor dust, mold and even insects such as cockroaches when over-stuffed with clothes, old newspapers, magazines and the like. It's surprising, in fact, just how much dust can find its way inside even when the doors have been tightly shut.

Make certain all clothing in closets has enough space to "breath". Every article should be on hangers. And it's not a bad idea to seal these articles in garment bags.

And don't get tricky with yourself by placing all the discards in the garage, attic or basement. They will eventually overwhelm you. Besides, it won't be a pretty sight whenever you have to face the prospect of cleaning out these areas.

---

✳ **Handy Hint:** Devote some of your excess items to a garage sale and make some extra money in the process.

---

One other way to clear out some of the clutter without eliminating it is to suspend certain usable items under cabinets or on walls. Yard and repair tools can be hung out of the way on a garage wall or partition. Coffee makers, can openers and the like can be hung below your kitchen cabinet. This will make it far easier to clean counter-tops and other surfaces where these objects have previously rested.

Another possibility to consider if you want to salvage some of your cherished dust-catchers is to make use of glass cases, like those used for trophy displays or entertainment centers. You can either equip existing cabinets or other enclosures with glass doors or purchase pre-built display cases. They're really quite a bargain. The objects will be visible but the dust will stay out.

---

❋ **Handy Hint:** Furniture itself can contribute to clutter if there is an overabundance of it. Keep rooms as simply furnished as possible. And try to arrange your furniture in a way that can be easily cleaned around with the mop or vacuum cleaner.

---

The important thing to remember is to find an appropriate place for everything you elect to keep and keep it there. But if it cannot be easily accommodated, eliminate it by tossing, selling, donating, or passing it on to a friend. You might ask yourself: is it really necessary to own a dozen pairs of shoes or a stack of magazines that are 10 years old? What about out-of-style clothes? And you certainly have no more use for medications that have expired, worn out tools, or outdated receipts. For those who want help in this endeavor, there are even on-line organizing services available. Just check the internet.

## Storage Solutions

For those who want to rescue some of their would-be dispelled articles, storage space in the home can be increased in a number of ways. Try installing drawers under beds. Mount caddies in the shower for shampoo and the like. Towel or knife racks can be placed under cabinets. Use the space under a built-in window seat as a chest for your children's toys. Use empty jars in the garage for nuts and bolts.

Outside storage in the form of a shed is another possibility. Such measure will help relieve your overflow. However, don't get caught sweeping your cleaning problems under the rug, as it were. These storage areas should not be used as a substitute for proper cleaning procedures.

Generally speaking, it's a good idea to store items you use most often waist level or higher. It's easier than bending down.

---

⊠ **Caution:** Always store potentially dangerous items such as medications and matches out of the reach of children.

---

Another thing to consider: hooks. They can be used to hang coats, belts or other such articles on the back of closet doors (provided the doors aren't the sliding variety). You can also use this strategy for hanging cups in cabinets. Another idea is to install tracks under shelves for storing wine glasses.

Consider placing items that have a higher potential to make a mess, such as honey jars or vegetable oil bottles, on sheets of aluminum foil in your cabinet. It is a whole lot easier to discard the foil than to clean the shelf.

---

❋ **Handy Hint:** Here's an idea from Donna Smallin, author of "Unclutter Your Home" in regard to storing plastic grocery bags. Cut a 3-inch hole in the side of a plastic milk carton and stuff the bags inside. You'd be surprised how many the jug will hold.

---

## Cover Yourself

That is: cover certain items around the house when not in use. Keep piano covers closed. Use plastic covers for computer printers and slipcovers for upholstery. Even baseboard heaters and wall radiators, often overlooked as objects that accumulate dust, should be covered in the summertime.

Upholstery slipcovers are especially handy since sofas and chairs collect such a large amount of dust. These slipcovers are available in a wide range of colors and styles. They can be removed and cleaned in the washing machine or shaken out in the backyard. In addition, they will take the abuse that kids and pets might offer rather than the furniture itself.

## Putting Pets in Their Place

The whole family certainly loves their pets, but animals can create a lot of extra work if they are allowed to roam indoors. The wisest decision is to leave them in their rightful domain—out-of-doors.

All right, so your children will never speak to you again if you even suggest the idea. Or maybe *your* heart melts every time you picture those adorable eyes in the harsh outdoors. Fortunately, there are some constructive measures you can take:

- Keep your pet groomed. It should be brushed 2 or 3 times a week—outside, of course, is best. The brush should be soft because stiff ones will scrape the skin and release more dander. And, as might be expected, long-haired animals require more attention in this respect. It is more difficult to remove the excess hair from them.

- Another idea is to wipe the pet down with a wet towel. This is a good way to remove much of the loose hair. Even a moist hand rubbed over a short-haired animal will pull out a surprising number of hairs.

- Regular baths are also in order to prevent dirt from being spread throughout the house. Dogs can often be enough of a problem when it comes to a bath, but cats are worse, unless they are very young. A good strategy is to give the animal a treat just before and just after washing it. Hopefully, that will condition it well enough to make your experience tolerable. It is well that a pet be shampooed at least every other week. This can remove not only most of the loose hair, but as much as 85% of the dander. Use of a veterinary shampoo is best, as the animal's sensitive skin is not designed for the harsher formulas produced for human scalps. Your pet's coat can even be made non-static by rinsing it with a solution of one teaspoon of fabric softener in a quart of water.

After the pet is bathed is the best time to wash its bedding. That way it will be easier to remember and the pet will start out fresh with a clean bed.

• To reduce scratching damage, keep claws trimmed.

• Provide a special place for your dog or cat, like a bed or pad that is clean and comfortable. If it is appealing, this will encourage the animal to spend more of its time there rather than on a chair, or rubbing against furniture. It is certainly easier to clean the hair from a pet's bed than to have to chase that hair down all over the house.

• If your pet already has a well-established favorite hangout that it insists on keeping, such as a chair in the living room, at least place some kind of a removable cover over it. That way it can be easily removed and laundered.

- Try to keep your pet off carpeting. Carpets will attract a lot of the hair and dander, as will upholstery.

- If you are dealing with a cat, make sure its litter box is kept clean. Whenever it gets too full, cats won't want to use it and will find another place to go—usually the most inconvenient place for its master to scrub. If you live in a conducive area, avoid kitty litter, which usually contains potent deodorants that might cause allergies, and train your cat to go outside. If you do use kitty litter, pour it into a metal pan rather than one made of plastic and change the litter frequently. Baking soda can be added to control odor. If odor is a particularly severe problem, consider changing your cat's diet.

- Secure your pet's food and water dishes. At least that way they won't get tipped over. And while you're at it, why not put an old towel under those dishes? It'll help you catch any spills or accidental overflows.

---

❋ **Handy Hint:** If a pet is kept indoors, its shedding is worse than normal because light has a bearing on the shedding process. In outside conditions, a dog or cat will only shed 2 times a year—in fall and late spring. If it remains inside, where electric lights are turned on at dark, the shedding will continue year round. So if shedding is too much of a problem to keep up with, and you want to use your lights, you will have to leave the pet outdoors.

## Controlling "Indoor Weather"

Ever wish you could turn off a rain storm that was spoiling a family picnic? You certainly would've been a big hit with the kids. But you know such a miracle is well beyond your ability.

However, controlling the "indoor weather" is a different proposition. Of course, it is done year round as a matter of routine, at least as far as temperature is concerned. But keep two things in mind. When the temperature is cooler, airborne dust is not as prevalent. More of it will be confined to surfaces, allowing you to get rid of larger amounts of it. So don't keep the thermostat setting any higher than you have to. Second, when the humidity level remains between 40 and 60%, not only will the amount of airborne dust decrease, but the proliferation of mold, dust mites, bacteria and viruses will be slowed down. You'll notice whenever the temperature moves out of the comfort range, but it's easy to neglect the indoor humidity. If you reside in a moist climate, such as in a coastal region, a dehumidifier should be considered if you don't already have one as part of your heating/cooling system.

> ❋ **Handy Hint:** You might want to consider investing is a hygrometer, a device that measures relative humidity. They are inexpensive and readily available.

Be especially wary of basements. They are notorious for contributing moisture to the air. Any water that accumulates in the ground around the house will press against basement walls, especially near the bottom where pressure is at its highest, and eventually work its way through cracks, gaps and joints.

Any imperfections should be patched to keep moisture outside. A good compound to employ is hydraulic cement, a quick-setting substance sold at paint and hardware stores, which expands on contact with water. It can even be used while water is seeping through.

To confirm the origin of a moisture problem, tightly tape a piece of aluminum foil to the basement wall when it is dry. When dampness recurs, if the side of the foil facing you is wet, the problem is condensation. But if the side that has been contacting the wall is moist, water is penetrating from outside.

Also inspect other areas in and around the house where unanticipated moisture could accumulate. Check window-mounted air conditioners for standing water and supply adequate drainage if needed. Make sure the insulation surrounding central air vents is intact. If any has come off, moisture can build up inside the vents. Check rainspouts to make certain an excess amount of water isn't building up too close to the foundation. If a problem of this nature exists, reroute the flow of water by using an extension or install concrete troughs. And don't hold still for a leaky roof.

It's also a good idea to check outdoor shrubbery. Hedges planted too close to outside walls can impede airflow and reduce evaporation in the lower extremities of the house. This holds especially true for walls that don't receive much sunlight. Trim back or remove any plants that are suspect.

During the day, keep drapes open so that condensed air won't form on the windows. Another way to minimize the creation and collection of moisture is to install double windows.

Don't forget to adequately insulate your home. Poorly insulated structures will admit moist air into the wall cavities. Even the small amount of air leaking through an inadequately sealed electrical outlet during the winter months will pull in more moisture than what can diffuse through 1,000 square feet of a typical plaster wall! And, of course, a poorly insulated structure will run up heating/cooling bills and cost you money.

---

✳ **Handy Hint:** Maintain a lower-than-average temperature in your home. While this is no substitute for cleaning, it will at least help somewhat in holding down the airborne particulate count—and cut heating costs in winter.

---

Another thing you'll want to control is smog. It may not be visible as such, and it might not technically qualify as smog, but the use of fireplaces results in a certain amount of soot and other debris (toxic hydrocarbons) that will adhere to walls, furniture, ceilings and everything else in the room. This is bad enough under normal conditions, but sometimes a change of air pressure will reverse the direction of air flow and create a big puff of smoke (known as a backdraft or downdraft). As it is, even when fireplaces are not in use at the moment, wind can sometimes blow out soot. Unless you have a flaming romance for this kind of heating device, you will be much better off abandoning it.

If you simply cannot give it up, make certain the damper is functioning properly, and keep it closed when the fireplace is not in use. Never close it, however, until the ashes cool after you have allowed flames to die, and always open it *before* lighting a fire. Also, installing glass doors across the front will contain a lot of the soot. Have the chimney as well as the fireplace cleaned at the end of every season.

---

⊠ **Caution:** The use of old newspapers as a fuel in a fireplace (or a wood stove, for that matter) is not advisable. This can create additional toxic vapors to your indoor atmosphere.

---

⊠ **Caution:** Never allow a fire to smolder. A fire that remains hot will contribute less to indoor air pollution.

---

One more major factor can contribute to this kind of pollution in your inside environment: smoking. It has been discovered that cigarette smoke can release anywhere from 1,500 to 3,000 different harmful chemicals. In addition to this it also expels heavy dust—not very helpful for whoever happens to be cleaning. You'd best trade your cigarettes for a "No Smoking" sign.

## Air Filtration

Air filtration is very important in keeping the air free of undesirable particles, as well as adding to the efficiency of the heating/cooling system and saving you money. Replace filters regularly. If they are of the washable variety, examine them at appropriate intervals and make sure to clean them when necessary.

Also understand that, when filters have aged, they can release bits of the material from which they are made. Fiberglass furnace filters, for instance, may eventually begin to disperse glass fibers into the air. This is another good reason for inspecting and maintaining your air filters.

---

※ **Handy Hint:** Air filters may be treated with oils, adhesives or the like to increase their ability to trap particles. But if you have one that is not, such as an untreated metal mesh filter, you can spray it with olive oil.

---

You might also want to consider installing charcoal filter pads to each of the room vents of central air systems. This will help keep the dust count down even more, but remember that they must be replaced when they get dirty.

Much more efficient passive filters intended to replace the conventional kind are also available for central heating and air conditioning systems. The best selection is a HEPA (High-Efficiency Particulate Air) filter. A HEPA filter is made from extremely thin glass fibers pressed into a pleated paper. HEPA filters too will have to be replaced regularly (according to manufacturer's instructions).

There are also electrostatic filters designed for central air systems, but a pre-filter is also required for capturing larger particles. Both the electrostatic filter and the pre-filter must be washed at appropriate intervals. It should also be said, though, that electrostatic filters release a small amount of ozone. Beware if you know you are sensitive to ozone.

## Don't Duck Out on Duct Cleaning

No matter what kind of a filter is used for your central heating and cooling system, it is good policy to have the air ducts professionally cleaned every few years. They can easily remain one of the most contaminated places in the house because they are so inaccessible for cleaning and such a large percentage of the matter in the air circulates through them. And if excess dust is thrown back into the air, it will settle in carpets, upholstery, draperies and the like to add to your cleaning chores.

---

⊠ **Caution:** In order to benefit properly from duct cleaning, carpets must also be clean or the ducts will more quickly become recontaminated because dust will be stirred up by foot traffic and pulled back in to the system. Then the central air system will blow it back out into the air. For a thorough job, your carpeting should be professionally steam-cleaned around the same time you are having the ducts cleaned. Better yet, remove carpeting and use hardwood floors.

---

Keeping air ducts clean will also increase the efficiency of your heating/cooling system, thereby saving you money.

## Portable Air Purifiers

Air purifiers can also help the cleaning cause. The small table models found in department stores and drug stores are the most economical way to go. They remove some of the airborne matter.

For a more thorough job, however, there are purifiers that use HEPA filters. The HEPA filter is customarily piggybacked with two other kinds of filters: a pre-filter for capturing larger particles (to protect the HEPA filter from becoming clogged) and an activated charcoal filter for absorbing certain odors. Purifiers using HEPA filters are capable of removing the vast majority of the foreign matter in the air. In fact, they meet rigid industrial standards and are utilized in such places as electronic chip manufacturing facilities and operating rooms.

Other portable devices for cleaning the air come in the form of electronic (or electrostatic) air cleaners. These portable units charge particles electronically and pull them out of the air, where they are deposited on a special plate. They are not, however, as efficient as HEPA filters and their efficiency tends to drop over time. In addition, they produce a small measure of ozone.

A similar kind of portable electronic air cleaner is a negative-ion generator. It generates negatively charged ions that intercept particles and pull them back to a filter in the unit. The generator, however, also emits ozone.

## Choosing a Vacuum Cleaner

There is no doubt that conventional vacuuming devices make the house look better, but dust will return on surfaces far too quickly to suit anyone who has charge of house cleaning. The reason for this is because some of the dust that is picked up is actually blown back out through the porous bag (the only means of exhaust the device possesses) to be redistributed into the air and once again settle on surfaces. And this process typically takes place within the hour. You might not notice it on surfaces quite that soon because the particles are so small, but as dust continues to accumulate under normal hustle-and-bustle, and is added to what's already present, it won't take very many days before surface dust will become evident again.

Anyone with doubts need only to turn on a conventional vacuum cleaner with a partially full bag and look closely while shining a light on the exhaust grill (the place around the bag where the warm air is rushing out). It is amazing what one can often see being expelled before even running the device across a carpet.

A better test still is to completely cover one side of a small index card or heavy piece of paper with double stick tape, and attach it to a portion of the exhaust area, making sure it is secure by placing more tape along the outside borders. (Don't cover the entire portion of the exhaust, however, or the air flow will be cut off.) Then try vacuuming part of a room. You won't believe what turns up on the tape.

As it is, the air flow of a conventional vacuum cleaner is weak anyway and many dust particles are left behind. The more packed the bag gets, the less-effective your cleaning job will be because the more the air flow will be reduced and, therefore, the less the suction will be. To get an idea of how much dirt remains on a carpet, if it is not attached, fold a loose corner of it over a piece of fresh white paper and tap the backing. Chances are your paper will not still be white.

If you continue to use a conventional vacuum cleaner, don't forget to follow the advice previously stated: change the bag out-of-doors, change it when only half full, clean the area around the bag before installing a fresh bag, and run the machine for at least 30 seconds before returning it to the house.

A non-electric portable sweeper (known to many as a carpet sweeper) can be used when one does not want to pull as much dust into the air. However, it is not quite as efficient as a powered device in picking up dirt. It too should be emptied outdoors and the inside compartment cleaned with a dust cloth.

There are other alternatives, however, that may be for you. Accessory filters are available that can be added to some conventional vacuum cleaners (the canister type, *e. g.*, the kind employing a hard outer shell), thereby reducing the number of particles they emit. They aren't designed to function, however, on upright machines, those that use a soft bag.

If you choose this route, remember that these filters require regular change or their purpose will be defeated. If a blockage occurs out of neglect, debris can be forced through the sides of the filter and the mechanism will lose suction. Also, in some instances, the motor could overheat.

Another option involves other types of vacuuming equipment, which perform better. One is a central vacuum system, which uses a network of ducts throughout the house that directs dirt to a unit usually mounted in the garage. It is a worthwhile device in that it deposits all the dirt somewhere else besides the interior of the home. But installing all the duct work that is required may very well be impractical as well as expensive for you. It's something to consider, however, if building a new home.

A number of other portable varieties are on the market that use a bag and filter combination, which are more efficient. Some models, known as bagless uprights, simply employ a HEPA filter. Just as with any vacuuming device, they must be maintained.

Another option is a portable unit whose operation depends upon a basin of water to trap the dirt. In this type of system, known to some as a water-trap vacuum cleaner, any and all water soluble material that is pulled in is absorbed by the swirling liquid. Air flow is never impeded because, since the water makes the device so efficient, there is no filter to become clogged. Furthermore, only pure air is released via the exhaust ports. Also, the emptying process is more efficient because one is dealing with dirty water, not the dry matter that can easily escape into the air and land on clothes and hair, and be picked up on shoes. Furthermore, since this is a water-base system, it can be used for wet pick up as well.

## Airing Out the House

Occasionally you might want to air out the house. But it is important to remember it should not be done under certain conditions. Always note the direction of the wind and watch for nearby activities that could be sending a high concentration of contaminants your way. Some examples are barbecuing, trash burning, yard mowing, road or parking lot resurfacing, pesticide spraying, or painting. Of course, one should never invite outdoor air inside during times of heavy pollution.

Generally, the best times to air out your home is early morning since the air will be fresher then, or just after a rain shower when particulate matter will have been washed from the air.

## Feathers that Fowl the Air

Watch out for deteriorating feather-stuffed items such as pillows, quilts, upholstery, mattresses and the like. Bits of matter from these articles can work their way loose and begin to ride the air only to settle someplace else you don't want it. Besides giving you something else to clean up, such particulate matter can cause hay fever, asthma, or other respiratory ailments when inhaled.

A quick fix for a feather pillow is to cover each side with a pillow case. This will help keep down the particle count. Mattresses as well as box springs can be wrapped in a dust-proof casing or plastic covering. In the end, however, it is a better policy to replace the worn out item.

## "Constructive" Activities Contributing to Dust

Beware hobbyists and workers. A number of activities impart their share of particulate matter. When filing, sanding, planing or drilling, the particulate count of the surrounding air quality zooms upward. Tiny bits of wood, metal, plastic or other material are readily released. This matter too can cause health problems as well as make your cleaning job harder. Wood dust from oak is especially bad about bringing on asthma attacks, although other kinds can be just as much of a concern. Plastic and metal dust can also be very harmful to the lungs.

Unless absolutely necessary, confine all such activity to a place beyond the confines of the house. The garage would probably be your first thought and, true, that is better than using the living quarters, but unless that garage is not attached to the house or there is no access from that point to the house, a lot of the debris in the air from such activities will sneak inside the house. It would be best to work out-of-doors when practical or devote an off-site workshop to the activity. The use of a filter mask while working is also a good idea.

## Seeing the Light

Another formidable object when it comes to dusting is the hanging light fixture, especially the chandelier. Recessed lighting is an attractive substitute, and it seems to be more the style these days anyway. The next best are ceiling lights that completely enclose the light bulb. Keep in mind, too, that lamps (whether the table or floor variety) are also difficult to clean around.

> ❋ **Handy Hint:** Don't forget about the light bulbs themselves. Unless they are well-sealed from the air, they're going to collect their share of dust. A damp cloth (after the bulb has cooled) is all you need.

## Localization

Another helpful idea is to keep the most frequently used and messiest items confined to one area of the house. For example, paper towel racks, storage shelves, trash containers and recycling bins can be grouped as close together as practical in the kitchen. This spot may get more heavily soiled because of the higher volume of traffic, but dirt will be concentrated there and not thinly spread more over the entire dwelling.

> ❋ **Handy Hint:** Use trash containers with foot pedals and attached lids. That way garbage odors will stay confined.

It will also be helpful to confine all of your seldom used items to one compartment. That way you'll only have to open that particular cabinet, closet or drawer on an occasional basis, which will give dust and dirt less of a chance to enter and accumulate.

Localizing can also come in another form. Try to confine you and your family's entrances and exits to one door. That way any debris that enters will tend to be confined to that area of the house.

## The Right Kind of Materials

Another thing to remember is that some materials used in the home are easier to keep clean than others. Some examples of hard to clean (*i. e.*, high-maintenance) surfaces are: porous countertops; floor coverings with indentations; ornate furniture; decorative pillows; blinds (particularly the horizontal variety); louvered doors; bed canopies; bunk beds; rough-textured ceilings; soft woods (such as fir or pine) or raw unfinished wood; flocked or uncoated wallpaper; soft, easily scratched plastics; long-napped carpeting; upholstery, heavy draperies, cotton velvets; and intricate handles and hardware.

Carpeting and upholstery can be especially bad because not only are these materials more of a challenge to maintain, but as they deteriorate, small bits of matter will break free and find their way into the air to eventually settle somewhere else.

You'll be better off if you stick to low-maintenance materials such as masonry (terrazzo, brick, concrete, stone or any similar substance bonded with mortar), glass, Formica (plastic laminate) or other hard plastics, ceramics or porcelain, finished hardwoods (such as oak, maple or walnut), rounded- or beveled-edged surfaces, stainless steel, and aluminum (as well as other metals).

You'll also be more efficient in cleaning when there are fewer kinds of surfaces grouped together in one area. As you well know by now, each requires separate care in order to be properly maintained. For instance, walls that contain wainscoting, wallpaper and a wood trim, in addition to a set of large mirrors, will require far more attention than mere unadorned paneled walls. This may be plainer to you, but that doesn't mean it isn't attractive.

And here's something else to consider: If you are having new plumbing fixtures installed, choose the kind with a single handle. Why have more obstacles there to clean around than necessary? Also bear in mind that deeper sinks will result in less splatter, and therefore less cleaning, just as suspended toilets are a better choice because there is no base to get dirty.

Another item that makes cleanup matters easier is the wire shoe rack. Wooden, plastic and other solid varieties accumulate dust. But airborne debris has less area to cling to wire racks—most of it simply falls through to the floor. And wire racks or shelving are a good idea in another respect. It beats moving individual pairs of shoes when cleaning closet floors. Wire shelving may also be used to store other articles and are beneficial because they furnish ventilation, and that means items stored on them for extended periods of time are less likely to fall victim to mildew. They are available in long strips that can be cut down to specifications.

There are also some materials that simply don't belong in certain areas of the home. For instance, easily marred walls and furniture have no place in a child's room. And carpeting should never be a part of the bathroom, kitchen or utility room because of the excess moisture present at these sites. A certain amount of shower or bath water inevitably splashes out of the tub, toilets have a way of running over sooner or later, washing machine hoses can spring leaks or become unattached, and no one can cook or use the refrigerator for very long without spilling something. This can rapidly transform carpeting into an excellent breeding ground for mildew, dust mites and bacteria. (Actually, carpeting is not such a good idea for kid's rooms either.)

On the other hand, some materials demand to be put in their proper places. There is no need for anything but an unfinished wall in the garage. Who would consider anything else but tile for the bathroom? And no kitchen should be without a backsplash behind the stove.

---

❋ **Handy Hint:** Make sure your backsplash runs as far up the wall as possible. Those greasy splashes do not always confine themselves to the lower areas. Any portion of the wall that is not covered is not only unprotected, but it will count as another kind of surface to clean.

---

## Maintenance Ratings of Some Typical Materials Used in the Home

### High-Maintenance

Bed Canopies
Blinds
Bunk Beds
Cotton Velvets
Decorative Pillows
Fancy Cabinets
Flocked or Uncoated Wallpaper
Floor Coverings with Indentations
Intricate Handles and Hardware
Long-Napped Carpeting
Louvered Doors
Ornate Furniture
Porous Counter-tops
Raw, Unfinished Wood
Rough-Textured Ceilings
Soft Woods
Soft, Easily-Scratched Plastics
Upholstery

### Low-Maintenance

Aluminum
Brick
Ceramics
Concrete
Finished Hardwoods
Glass
Glass Cases
Marble
Plastic Laminate (Formica) or other Hard Plastics
Porcelain
Rounded- and Beveled-Edged Surfaces
Stainless Steel
Stone
Terrazzo
Wire Shelving

## Discouraging Insects

Insects are anything but a welcome sight around the house when you are cleaning. But using pesticides—conventional pesticides, that is—can pose just as serious of a problem as harsh chemical cleaners. More often than not, in fact, these substances are far worse. And if you call in professional help you'll incur a big expense.

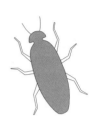

But just as with cleaning chemicals, there are a number of safe, inexpensive substitutes for eliminating insects. The following are suggested:

**Ants:** Red pepper, dried peppermint or paprika can be used. Just sprinkle in strategic spots. Also, honey and boric acid or borax thinly applied to small strips of paper can be effective. Jelly or jam can be substituted for honey. Initially this will attract them as they go after the sweet-tasting substance, but they will carry some of it back to the queen and eventually they will disappear. Another idea is to plant peppermint or pansies around doors and windows outside. They serve as good repellents.

**Roaches and silverfish:** Boric acid is effective for these insects. For roaches, sprinkle in corners, along baseboards, or whereever they are noticed. When dealing with silverfish, since they hold such a remarkable affinity for paper, mix the boric acid with flour and sugar and place on strips of paper. In addition, plain baking soda is toxic to roaches. Just mix with an equal amount of sugar and distribute. You may have to repeat this process for several weeks in order to kill newly hatched roaches. Also, roach traps that contain natural food bait and no insecticides can be used, not only for roaches, but for a number of other crawling insects.

**Beetles:** To prevent these insects from getting into foodstuffs, store all vulnerable items, such as grains and flours, in a cool spot in tightly sealed containers. Place a bay leaf in each container.

**Fleas:** To discourage these pests, add brewer's yeast to your pet's food. It will give an odor to the animal's skin that the fleas detest. Pine needles placed in and around dog houses will also help. Another effective measure is to salt the crevices of the dog house. Of course, animal bedding should be washed frequently, preferably with a mild, non-phosphate, biodegradable soap. And don't neglect your pet's nutritional requirements. If a dog or cat should fall ill, it will be more prone to attack by fleas. Add raw meat and a mixture of raw vegetables to the diet. Check with your veterinarian for details.

**Moths:** For a mothball substitute, try cedar wood shavings, blocks or balls. Also, for apparel that is to be stored for lengthy periods, wrap in paper and freeze a week or so prior to storing. Of course, it is well to wash or brush frequently worn clothing regularly. The insect and its eggs are fragile and cannot take activity.

**Flies:** These flying pests can be repelled with basil plants. Grow them around doors and windows. If necessary, hang homemade flypaper (made by applying a thin coat of honey to yellow paper) or use outdoor "zappers". Flies can also be repelled by hanging clusters of cloves in the affected area.

**Mosquitos:** Grow basil plants around doors and windows or use outdoor "zappers". The breeding of mosquitos should be prevented by emptying any stagnant water on the premises.

Of course, it goes without saying that many pest problems in the home can be reduced or even eliminated by maintaining clean habits in the first place. Ants are attracted to sugar and grease. Roaches adore all kinds of food remnants, as do flies. And, needless to say, everyone knows what can be the consequences of inviting in a flea-infested animal.

---

⊠ **Caution:** Make no mistake. Although it releases no toxic vapors, boric acid is still a poison. Do not ingest this substance or allow children or pets access to it.

---

To discourage insect's entry, caulk around doors and windows. Also, examine any gaps between pipes and stuff with steel scrubbing pads.

## A Word about Rodents

Mice can be dealt with by putting mousetraps to work. Put them along baseboards or in corners. Mice will be more likely to find them there because they seldom roam in open spaces. It is customary to bait them with cheese, but you can get more creative. Bacon or chocolate can usually also be used. If one bait fails, try another. To prevent their entry, try to locate the entrance sites and block those with an enduring substance such as steel wool or metal.

Also, a poison can be concocted that poses less hazard to children and pets. Make a mixture of one part flour, one part plaster of paris, and a dash of cocoa powder and sugar and sprinkle in areas where mice are sure to find it. This also works for rats if preferred over rat traps.

## Plants to the Rescue

Plants? What do they possibly have to do with cleaning the house? They won't do anything about keeping down dust and dirt, but they deserve a word here. Many varieties (via their respiration process) are capable of ridding the air of certain chemicals that might be lingering there. NASA research on air contamination has proven it. For a measure of protection against formaldehyde, furnish some of your rooms with spider plants, golden pathos, rubber plants, philodendrons or snake plants. If there is room, even fig trees can help the cause. In addition, chrysanthemums, gerbera daisies and English ivy are especially efficient at reducing toxins such as benzene. For general air purification, try any of the above, if not aloe vera, banana trees, Chinese evergreen, dracaena, mother-in-law's tongue, peace lily or reed palm.

Plants are more effective at absorbing air-laden chemicals in enclosed areas.

Water them sparingly, however, since a lot of extra moisture can give rise to mold.

---

⊠ **Caution:** Don't depend solely on plants to clear the air in extreme cases. They will eventually do their job, but if you are painting, varnishing, or involved in any project in which strong chemicals are used, or if you have had a serious chemical spill, you will need to supply the house with some quick ventilation. Better yet, don't even use potent substances inside unless it is absolutely necessary.

---

**A List of Plants that Effectively Clean the Air**

Aloe Vera
Banana Trees
Chinese Evergreen
Chrysanthemums
Dracaena
English Ivy
Fig Trees
Gerberaes
Golden Pathos
Philodendrons
Mother-In-Law's Tongue
Peace Lily
Reed Palm
Rubber Plants
Snake Plants
Spider Plants

## Safe Air Deodorizers

There are times when an air deodorizer becomes necessary. A number of simple, safe and inexpensive materials can be put to use for this purpose.

One of these substances is probably already in your refrigerator. It's baking soda, the easiest and probably the most accessible. For best results in removing stale air, pour some of it into open containers and place them in strategic spots around the house. This works especially well in closets.

Vinegar can also help in this respect. Again, open containers should be placed in appropriate spots. This is particularly effective for areas that reek of paint, glue, sealants and the like. In addition, you can combine a tablespoon of vinegar and a cup of water in a pan and bring to a boil.

And there's another item especially effective for absorbing fresh paint odors. Believe it or not, it's hay. Just place a handful in a bucket of warm water and leave overnight.

Still, another idea for deodorizing the air is charcoal. It's used as an auxiliary filter for electric air purifiers (as well as for water filtration). This substance gives the air an unmistakably clean aroma and it is very efficient. If you can locate small bags of charcoal granules, like those used in radon testing (or simply put to use a few blocks from your backyard barbecue grill), you'll be successful at eliminating any unwanted odors.

Essential oils also fill the bill. They are more concentrated and last longer than artificial fragrances. And not only do they offer pleasing aromas, university and medical studies have found that they are an excellent disinfectant! You can use rosewood, lemon, orange, frankincense, basil, oregano or clove, just to name a few—or try any combination you desire. Just add a few drops to a spray bottle and dilute with water (preferably distilled water). Inquire at your local health food store for therapeutic Grade A oils.

And try this one on for size. Don't just throw away used citrus rinds. Toss them in a pot of water and simmer them a while. Or try substituting 2 tablespoons of ground cinnamon.

---

❋ **Handy Hint:** Deposit a drop of vanilla flavoring or natural essential oil such as mint on a light bulb and turn it on.

---

**Safe Air Deodorizers**

| Name | Suggested Uses |
|------|----------------|
| Baking Soda | Refrigerators, Closets |
| Charcoal | General |
| Cinnamon | General |
| Citrus Rinds | General |
| Essential Oils | General |
| Hay | Fresh Paint Odors |
| Vinegar | Fresh Paint Odors |
| Vanilla Flavoring | General |

## Other Considerations

Always use placemats when eating. They're much easier to keep clean. Using trays also helps. For the same reason, it's a good idea to cover the floor under your children's chair, especially high chairs, with rubber matting.

A crib can be layered with several sheets and waterproof pads for quicker changes.

Cutting boards can be placed in the dishwasher just like the dishes.

A blender or food processor can be cleaned by placing some dishwashing soap in it and filling halfway with warm water. Cover and turn on the switch, then rinse and repeat as necessary.

In essence, it is obviously worthwhile to lighten your household cleaning burden as much as possible while keeping the indoor air fresh and inviting in the least expensive manner. This will encourage you to keep up with your household cleaning chores. Just several small investments, a few sacrifices and a little organization will go a long way.

## Conclusion

Cleaning is still a largely unwanted, never-ending, time consuming job no matter how you slice it. But in maintaining a clean home, you'll feel a lot better for your family and yourself. You'll also be discouraging insects, rodents and germs, thereby lessening the potential of toxic pesticide use and decreasing the chances that you will succumb to infection. In addition, you will be playing a big part in preserving your property. It will also provide a happier environment for everyone. And if household costs are kept down, all the better. Where there is neatness and cleanness—and more saved dollars, there are more cheerful dispositions. Who knows. You might even draw a few compliments!